D0083138

From Famine
to Fast Food

From Famine to Fast Food

NUTRITION, DIET, AND CONCEPTS OF HEALTH AROUND THE WORLD

Ken Albala, Editor

GREENWOOD

AN IMPRINT OF ABC-CLIO, LLC
Santa Barbara, California • Denver, Colorado • Oxford, England

Library of Congress Cataloging-in-Publication Data

From famine to fast food : nutrition, diet, and concepts of health around the world / Ken Albala, editor.

   p. ; cm.

Includes bibliographical references and index.

ISBN 978–1–61069–743–9 (alk. paper) — ISBN 978–1–61069–744–6 (ebook) I. Albala, Ken, 1964– editor of compilation. [DNLM: 1. Nutritional Status—Encyclopedias—English. 2. Cultural Characteristics—Encyclopedias—English. 3. Diet—Encyclopedias—English. 4. World Health—Encyclopedias—English. QU 13]

RA645.N87

363.803—dc23   2014000623

ISBN: 978–1–61069–743–9
EISBN: 978–1–61069–744–6

18 17 16 15 14   1 2 3 4 5

This book is also available on the World Wide Web as an eBook.
Visit www.abc-clio.com for details.

Greenwood
An Imprint of ABC-CLIO, LLC

ABC-CLIO, LLC
130 Cremona Drive, P.O. Box 1911
Santa Barbara, California 93116-1911

This book is printed on acid-free paper ∞

Manufactured in the United States of America

Contents

Introduction

We live in a world of shocking inequalities of wealth. That some people can overeat to the detriment of their health while others go hungry is the central paradox of modernity. That malnutrition can persist in countries where the silos are overflowing with grain, that junk food and fast food can flourish in the most nutrient deprived places on earth is simply inexcusable.

Inequality is as old as civilization itself. According to philosopher John Locke, when labor is congealed into imperishable goods, humans can rightfully claim to possess such goods as property. In other words, no one can own all the fruit on an apple tree, which would otherwise spoil, unless it is preserved in a form such as jelly that is owned as property. Jean-Jacques Rousseau added that as long as there has been property, wealth can be accumulated and the labor of one human can be purchased or coerced into service by another. This was the origin of social classes, haves and have-nots, wealthy and poor nations, the well fed and the hungry.

Barring natural disaster or crop failure, the unequal distribution of resources suggests that hunger is largely the by-product of civilization itself. History provides incontrovertible examples of this essential fact—whether it was grain diverted to higher-paying markets during the Irish Potato Famine, or rural populations in Central America and Africa goaded into growing monoculture crops like coffee or bananas for international commodity markets while indigenous and nutritious foods were neglected, or even in our own backyard as inner cities bereft of grocery stores become virtual food deserts and people are forced to feed at convenience stores or subsist on fast food. That means, counter to our intuition, hunger is not always the result of natural disasters but of systemic problems stemming from the way we grow, process, and distribute food.

Hungry people are also unruly. Given the threat of unrest and violence from the starving populations, ruling elites have also routinely provided solutions to the problem of hunger: handing out bread in ancient Rome, fixing prices and wages in medieval Europe, or forcefully redistributing land and trying to farm it collectively as happened in Stalinist Russia, which led to one of the world's most disastrous famines, leaving 10 million people dead. There is no doubt that for every government-sponsored public welfare scheme, there is another example of hunger and malnutrition caused directly by state policy. War is of course the greatest instigator of famine; the catastrophe in Darfur is only one recent example.

Hunger and malnutrition also derive not from intentional policy decisions, but from systemic problems in distribution and trade—that is, not the actions of individuals per se, but the ordinary functions of a food system that routinely denies certain people access to food while others are given free rein to seek personal profit. One example will suffice. In the wake of independence following World War II, India sought to modernize its agriculture. New technologies were imported—mechanized tractors, irrigation systems, chemical fertilizers, and hybrid crops—which offered the promise of bounty. All of these innovations were hailed as a Green Revolution. Yet instead of the traditional pattern of small diversified farms providing an array of crops ideally suited to local conditions and grown with indigenous knowledge, huge monoculture mechanized farms growing food for export prevailed. Only the wealthiest of farmers could afford machines, fuel, expensive management techniques, and expensive seeds, which had to be purchased from suppliers rather than saved from the previous year's crop. These factors only widened the social divide, creating a landless impoverished class, even greater insecurity, and vulnerability to chronic malnutrition, disease, and outright famine—especially given the great demand on water supplies to irrigate intensively farmed crops, not to mention environmental degradation due to runoff and poisoning of the soil. In other words, what seemed like progress left greater poverty in its wake even though overall production of food increased.

The typical humanitarian response to such crises has taken the form of charity as either an act of pious benevolence, moral obligation, or simply guilt-induced coins tossed into the cup of the indigent. While such charity certainly has its place, critics have claimed that people really need jobs, and that it is better to teach them to fish than give them a fish, which only feeds them for a day. But it does not feed them at all if the pond is poisoned.

There have been many proposed solutions to these inequities, often going beyond voluntary contributions and government-sponsored programs.

The chapters of this encyclopedia will describe the vast divergence of situations across the globe, which will suggest not only that there are no simple solutions but that no one solution fits for every location. Health and nutrition policies must be tailor-made for every nation, every family, and every individual.

The two problems we face globally, hunger and obesity, are actually two sides of the same coin. It is much more complicated than some people having a lot to eat and others having little. For example, in the United States the states with the highest rates of obesity are also among the poorest. In 2011, Mississippi led with 34.5 percent; Alabama weighed in with 33 percent; West Virginia was right behind, followed by Tennessee, Kentucky, and Louisiana. Obviously, there is a wide range of income levels in all these states and it may not be fair to categorize people by state, but in general obesity rates go down dramatically as median income rises. That is, the more money you have the less likely you are to be obese, which also revealingly correlates with level of education. Conversely, the poorer and less educated, the greater the incidence of obesity.

The methods of collecting these data have been criticized as well as the very definition of obesity now in use, based on body mass index. If you redefine obesity to be more inclusive, of course rates will rise—and of course the national obsession with the obesity epidemic has been pandered to by the weight loss industry, which makes more profit if it can convince more people to buy its products and try its therapies. These quibbles aside, there is no doubt that we are becoming a heavier nation and that there is a strong correlation between size and class. This is a situation unprecedented in history.

This situation stems not from a dearth of food, but in fact from relatively cheap food and a glut of a particular type of food—for the most part mass manufactured, loaded with salt, fat, and sugar, and sold under the banner of being quick, easy, and convenient. In this category we should place not only fast food and what is served in most franchised restaurants in the United States, but also much of what appears in supermarkets as convenience food in cans or the freezer section—often ironically marketed with explicit health claims. Or to put it more plainly, when hamburgers, soda, and snack foods are cheaper than fresh produce, people will naturally eat more of them, unless they have the expendable income and social values that dictate otherwise.

In recent years some politicians have suggested a so-called Twinkie Tax, or tax on any food deemed unhealthy. Presumably, the higher price will provide a disincentive to buy too much and added tax revenues could be spent on health education. Many researchers have proposed a tax on sugar and products containing it. In fact such a tax would merely take money and food out of the mouths of people who buy these products.

As for education, we have seen the first lady of the United States, Michelle Obama, sponsor various antiobesity programs, which do little more than advise people to get more exercise, but they do not focus on the quality of food at all, thanks to the lobbying of various food industries who fear their revenues may decrease if they are targeted as "bad foods." In any case, does it make sense to promote health and nutrition education while at the same time tax dollars support the companies that grow the corn that is made into high-fructose corn syrup, or the soy that becomes the oil that is used to make junk food? The state with one hand facilitates the prevalence of junk food and with the other advises us not to eat it.

But what does obesity have to do with hunger, and how can hunger be a problem if there are rising obesity rates? A closer look at the bottom tiers of the social strata in the United States will provide a good example. In 2012, 15.1 percent of Americans fell below the poverty line, which is defined as an income of about $22,000 for a family of four. That accounts for 42.6 million people, with a high percentage of women and children, and particularly people of color. That translates into a full 15 percent of Americans living with year-round food insecurity, which does not account for those with occasional insecurity due to job loss or other misfortune. There are different ways to measure food insecurity, which is not necessarily the same thing as chronic hunger; but it should be evident that while a certain segment of the population in the United States (about 30%) has the wherewithal to overeat, another significant segment in poverty (15%) falls below that threshold. This means nearly half the population constitutes a lower class, despite the fact that most Americans like to think of themselves as in the middle class.

Hunger and obesity are two sides of the same coin because these two segments, the 30 percent of obese and 15 percent of food insecure, are often in exactly the same places geographically. They are largely in rural economically depressed areas and inner cities. Or to put it more plainly, those who are able to live on fast food and junk food often live side by side with those who suffer malnutrition and hunger. These are two radically opposite physical effects from the same social causes. This pattern is replicated elsewhere around the globe as well.

If this indeed is a systemic problem rather than simply the lack of a decent safety net, then we need to look at the entire way food is grown, processed, marketed, and sold to find viable solutions. One brief example will illustrate this point. Consider a soybean grown in Missouri. That bean is planted on an enormous farm that grows nothing but soybeans. It is intensively culti-vated, which means the bulk of costs derive from fuel for tractors, chemicals to maintain pests, fertilizers to stimulate growth, and of course water to irri-gate. The largest cost, however, is to purchase the seeds from the corporation that owns the patent on the technology with which they were genetically modified. Ironically, this soybean is not eaten as food in its natural state. Mature soybeans do not taste very good; they are mostly used as cattle feed or in food processing. Let us follow the soybean to the point where it is pressed with chemical solvents to make vegetable oil, then processed into soy lecithin—a thickener you find in ice cream and baked goods—then vegetable protein that goes into vegetarian hotdogs, and a whole slew of soy-derived chemicals, flavorings additives, and stabilizers that can be described as "natural" on a label because they come from a living organism. There are no federal regulations in the United States regarding the use of the word "natural." All these products go into junk food, which is aggressively marketed to the public. It is fairly cheap, requires no preparation, lasts on the shelf indefinitely, and is consumed with consequences that nutritionists insist are dire. This is a situation being replicated around the world.

Speaking of the entire globe, the data here are a little more startling than the 15 percent poverty rate in the United States. According to UNICEF, 80 percent of chronically malnourished children live in 24 of the poorest countries in the world. They account for 178 million children. In Sub-Saharan Africa this is 28 percent of the population under five years of age. In Southern Asia it is 46 percent. Chronic malnutrition means lack of nutrients during pregnancy and the first two years of life, which leads to irre-versible detrimental effects on the body and brain development. These include stunted growth, problems with eyesight, impaired cognitive develop-ment, as well as diseases such as pellagra, beri beri, scurvy, and rickets. To be more specific, vitamin A deficiency, defined as less than 300 micrograms per person per day, is highest in countries like Bangladesh, Burkina Faso, Cambodia, and other adjacent countries. This can lead to Xerophthalmia or night blindness or in extreme cases total blindness in 250,000 to 500,000 children each year, half of which die within the next year.

The greatest source of vitamin A is liver, but after that dandelion greens, broccoli and kale, carrots, spinach, and sweet potatoes. So the question is why these children are no longer eating green vegetables—which have been for millennia central in their diets.

In many places around the world, people produce commodities for export—coffee, chocolate, and sugar—which do not provide sustenance.

These are the legacy of the colonial era, and while they can produce great wealth for the companies that purchase, distribute, and process these goods (often into junk food), they leave farmers elsewhere in the world highly dependent on the fluctuations of international trade. If the price of coffee drops a few cents per pound, then they can be devastated. More importantly, these same countries are no longer growing the range and extent of fresh vegetables and produce they once did—those leafy greens, which were grown in small garden plots or foraged but now have to be purchased with meager wages made from working on coffee plantations.

As for coffee production itself, there do exist companies that promote fair trade, which guarantees decent wages and working conditions and fair prices for these commodities. But by the time they get to affluent consumers elsewhere, they become an expensive luxury affordable only to those with the ideological commitment to support them. It is certainly not enough to drive a systemic change when most people buy ordinary coffee and chocolate.

Critics have suggested that instead of buying cheap bulk coffee and then handing out aid to reduce hunger around the world, or trying to get these people to grow genetically modified golden rice, which is supposed to supply the recommended requirement of vitamin A, what if that money were used to encourage people to grow their own food on small, diversified farms? This would include those leafy greens grown historically, which could in turn be marketed locally. Counterarguments insist that this would require a major step away from the process of globalization, that it would mean real hardship for the companies that sell coffee—and in fact the price would rise dramatically for us. Ultimately at stake here is not the price of coffee, but independence in indigenous food production, what food scholars call food sovereignty. In these cases hunger and deprivation is not the result of natural causes, but of accidental effects stemming from the food system itself.

Another major source of disjuncture occurs when nutritional scientists and dieticians informed by the latest findings seek to make recommendations to improve diet that fall of deaf ears because of ingrained habits, indigenous systems of thinking about health, or simply a failure to accommodate these recommendations into long-standing culinary preferences. The classic historic example occurred when Italian immigrants first arrived in the United States and were told to abandon their spicy vegetable- and pasta-centered, garlic-laden diet in favor of what was deemed to be more nutritious meat and potatoes. This plan thankfully backfired. But in more serious cases, we find powdered milk intended to supplement infant diets, but instead being used to whitewash houses in Africa. There are surplus items like peanut butter sent as relief that never get eaten, or simply a general failure to account for the way traditional foodways serve as medicine in so many cultures throughout the world.

Habits die hard for a very good reason; they are often well adapted to the environment and material circumstances much better than mass-produced Western foods. This encyclopedia intends to close this gap in understanding by situating indigenous knowledge about food and health into the overall picture, and recognizing that aggressively seeking to change people's foodways is not only very difficult but usually not desirable either. Religious strictures, taboos, and ingrained preferences linked to festive occasions and traditions are yet other factors that must be taken seriously; and they have a much greater impact on food and health than is generally recognized, so they too are given coverage here.

This encyclopedia is divided by continent and then alphabetically by nation, though in many cases regions are covered (such as central Asia or sections of the United States), and in some cases individual groups are covered due to their unique diets, such as the Maasai and Hmong. The encyclopedia also provides basic statistical information concerning demographic trends, life expectancy, expenditure on health care, as well as obesity and malnourishment rates. These hard data correlate with the more specific details about the eating habits and diet of each country. A variety of recipes showcasing traditional foods from a variety of countries have also been included to augment the main text. The overall intention is to suggest ways that our thinking about alleviating hunger and malnutrition will evolve beyond the simple handout or dietary supplement. This encyclopedia provides the details that will help us make informed policy decisions that can be applied to the radically different situations that prevail in countries around the world.

Ken Albala
University of the Pacific

Africa

Algeria

Population: 38,087,812 (July 2013 est.)
Population Rank: 34th
Population Growth Rate: 1.9% (2013 est.)
Life Expectancy at Birth: 76.18 years (2013 est.)
Health Expenditures: 3.9% of GDP (2011)
People with Access to Safe Drinking Water: 83% of population (2010 est.)
Average Daily Caloric Consumption: 3,110
Adult Obesity Rate: 16% (2008)
Underweight Children under Age 5: 3.7% (2005)

In some regions of Algeria, olive oil is highly prized for its purported medicinal value as a cure-all for minor ailments such as indigestion, headaches, and irritated skin. Gently heated olive oil is rubbed directly onto the skin to treat problem areas. Folk remedies also include herbal infusions. For example, in the Kabylie, water infused with fresh mint is believed to be a digestive aid with antispasmodic and antinausea properties. Proper digestion is considered very important; certain foods are eaten or avoided to prevent upset stomach.

Islamic culture places great emphasis on maintaining good health through proper personal hygiene and dietary habits. Ablution (ritual cleansing) is performed before each of the five daily prayers of Islam, and food is eaten with the right hand only; the left hand is reserved for matters of personal hygiene. Foods are either *haram* (prohibited) or *halal* (permitted). Haram foods include alcohol and other intoxicants; pork and products derived from pork such as gelatin; and blood, including meat that has not been completely drained of blood. Animals must be slaughtered according to *zabiha*, the prescribed Islamic methods for ritual slaughter, to be considered halal. All plant-based foods are halal.

Susan Ji-Young Park

Further Reading

Çelik, Zeynep, Julia Clancy-Smith, and Frances Terpak. *Walls of Algiers: Narratives of the City through Text and Images*. Seattle: University of Washington Press, 2009.

Rodinson, Maxime, A. J. Arberry, and Charles Perry. *Medieval Arab Cookery*. Devon, UK: Prospect Books, 2001.

Zaouali, Lilia. *Medieval Cuisine of the Islamic World: A Concise History with 174 Recipes*. Translated by M. B. DeBevoise. Berkeley: University of California Press, 2007.

Angola

Population: 18,565,269 (July 2013 est.)
Population Rank: 59th
Population Growth Rate: 2.78% (2013 est.)
Life Expectancy at Birth: 54.95 years (2013 est.)
Health Expenditures: 3.5% of GDP (2011)
People with Access to Safe Drinking Water: 51% of population (2010 est.)
Average Daily Caloric Consumption: 1,950
Adult Obesity Rate: 6.4% (2008)
Underweight Children under Age 5: 15.6% (2007)

The foods that are the mainstays of the traditional Angolan diet are manioc prepared in many ways (including the leaves of the plant), palm oil, peanuts, beans, rice, okra, hot chili peppers, sweet potatoes, bananas, corn, cashews, coconut, dried or fresh fish, dried or fresh beef, pork, and chicken. A majority of the Angolan population is considered to be underfed. So it is rare to find obesity. Given that 70 percent of the population lives in poverty and over half are unemployed, hunger is a serious problem. People living in the coastal areas eat a lot of seafood; in the southwest herders live primarily on dairy products and meat; and farmers consume their produce of maize, sorghum, cassava, and other crops. Gathering firewood and water in some rural areas requires a great deal of energy.

Medical care is not available everywhere despite government efforts. In rural areas clinics lack staff and basic equipment, and thus most people rely on traditional healers whose practice depends largely on herbal remedies. In the larger cities Angolans have better access to public health care at hospitals and clinics. There are also hospitals specifically to treat women's and children's illnesses. Angola recently appointed a regional director to the World Health Organization to oversee the fight against HIV/AIDS and other infectious diseases. The director will also work to provide better-quality health care to all citizens and to ensure better coordination of tracking diseases. Doctors of traditional medicine are also working with government approval to broaden their reach to people in the interior and introduce the use of medicinal plants as cures for some sicknesses.

Cherie Y. Hamilton

Muamba de Galinha (Angolan-Style Chicken)

Serves 8

4 lb boneless chicken thighs
2 large onions, minced
¾ c vegetable oil
2 large cloves garlic, chopped
1 bay leaf
½ to ¾ c palm oil, or half palm oil and half vegetable oil
4 fresh chili peppers (jindungo), chopped and seeded
1 lb pumpkin or butternut squash, peeled and cubed
1 lb okra, trimmed and cut in half if large
3 tbsp lemon juice
1 tsp salt

Cut the chicken thighs in half, and place them in a large pot with the onions, vegetable oil, garlic, and bay leaf over medium heat. Stir to mix the ingredients well. Cook for 20 minutes, or until the chicken is tender and the vegetables have formed a sauce, adding a little water from time to time to keep the dish from drying out.

Add the palm oil, peppers, pumpkin, okra, lemon juice, and salt. Cook over low heat for 15 minutes to allow seasonings to permeate the sauce. Serve hot in a large serving dish.

Further Reading

Hamilton, Cherie Y. *Cuisines of Portuguese Encounters*. New York: Hippocrene Books, 2008.

Hamilton, Russell G., and Cherie Y. Hamilton. "Caruru and Calulu, Etymologically and Socio-gastronomically." *Callaloo: A Journal of African Diaspora Arts and Letters* 30, No. 1 (2007): 338–42.

Benin

Population: 9,877,292 (July 2013 est.)
Population Rank: 89th
Population Growth Rate: 2.81% (2014 est.)
Life Expectancy at Birth: 60.67 years (2013 est.)
Health Expenditures: 4.6% of GDP (2011)
People with Access to Safe Drinking Water: 75% of population (2010 est.)
Average Daily Caloric Consumption: 2,510
Adult Obesity Rate: 6% (2008)
Underweight Children under Age 5: 20.2% (2006)

During the Socialist period (1972–91) the government encouraged rural development and favored agricultural initiatives, and the country is self-sufficient in food production. Almost half of the population is involved in some form of agriculture. An internal system of trade still functions and has the ability to ensure food distribution from one area to another. However, the lack of rural infrastructure means that intermittent food shortages are faced by about 900,000 people, mostly in the hard-to-reach northern parts of the country.

Jessica B. Harris

Further Reading

Bay, Edna G. *Wives of the Leopard: Gender, Politics, and Culture in the Kingdom of Dahomey.* Charlottesville: University of Virginia Press, 1998.

Harris, Jessica B. *The Africa Cookbook: Tastes of a Continent.* New York: Simon and Schuster, 1998.

Burkina Faso

Population: 17,812,961 (July 2013 est.)
Population Rank: 60th
Population Growth Rate: 3.06% (2013 est.)
Life Expectancy at Birth: 54.43 years (2013 est.)
Health Expenditures: 6.5% of GDP (2011)

People with Access to Safe Drinking Water: 79% of population (2010 est.)
Average Daily Caloric Consumption: 2,670
Adult Obesity Rate: 2.3% (2008)
Underweight Children under Age 5: 26% (2009)

African ideas of healthy eating are very different from Western ones. Possibly due to food shortages in the past, people eat as much as they can. Fatness equals good health, life force, and wealth and is an appreciated feature. People who become rich will initially start eating larger quantities of fattening foods. They will add extra foods to the communal meal and go for particularly rich breakfasts and several daytime snacks. With time, the same people might become more health conscious and start buying better-quality ingredients instead of simply doubling the quantity of their intake. In urban areas people are becoming more weight conscious, and some women talk about reducing fat in their food intake. However, since oil is a cherished ingredient and communal cooking does not consider special needs, those who wish to follow a special diet need to prepare their food themselves. This requires both time and money and is thus often not an option for many people. When people are unwell, meat soup and tô are considered as strength-giving foods. Tô is believed to be more easily digested than rice and thus more suitable for someone who is frail and ailing.

Liza Debevec

Further Reading

Debevec, Liza. "Family Meals, Sharing and Hierarchy in a West-African Town." In *Nurture: The Proceedings of Symposium on Food and Cookery*, edited by Richard Hosking, 66–77. Bristol, UK: Footwork Press, 2003.

Freidberg, Susanne. "French Beans of the Masses: A Modern Historical Geography of Food in Burkina Faso." *Journal of Historical Geography* 29, No. 3 (2003): 445–63.

Osseo-Asare, Fran. *Food Culture in Sub-Saharan Africa*. Westport, CT: Greenwood Press, 2005.

Central Africa

Cameroon

Population: 20,549,221 (July 2013 est.)
Population Rank: 58th
Population Growth Rate: 2.04% (2013 est.)
Life Expectancy at Birth: 55.02 years (2013 est.)

Health Expenditures: 5.2% of GDP (2011)
People with Access to Safe Drinking Water: 77% of population (2010 est.)
Average Daily Caloric Consumption: 2,260
Adult Obesity Rate: 10.3% (2008)
Underweight Children under Age 5: 16.6% (2006)

Central African Republic (CAR)

Population: 5,166,510 (July 2013 est.)
Population Rank: 117th
Population Growth Rate: 2.14% (2013 est.)
Life Expectancy at Birth: 50.9 years (2013 est.)
Health Expenditures: 3.8% of GDP (2011)
People with Access to Safe Drinking Water: 67% of population (2010 est.)
Average Daily Caloric Consumption: 1,960
Adult Obesity Rate: 3.5% (2008)
Underweight Children under Age 5: 28% (2006)

Democratic Republic of the Congo (DRC)

Population: 75,507,308 (July 2013 est.)
Population Rank: 19th
Population Growth Rate: 2.54% (2013 est.)
Life Expectancy at Birth: 56.14 years (2013 est.)
Health Expenditures: 8.5% of GDP (2011)
People with Access to Safe Drinking Water: 45% of population (2010 est.)
Average Daily Caloric Consumption:1,590
Adult Obesity Rate: 1.7% (2008)
Underweight Children under Age 5: 28.2% (2007)

Equatorial Guinea

Population: 704,001 (July 2013 est.)
Population Rank: 166th
Population Growth Rate: 2.58% (2013 est.)
Life Expectancy at Birth: 63.12 years (2013 est.)
Health Expenditures: 4% of GDP (2011)
People with Access to Safe Drinking Water: 43% of population (2000 est.)
Average Daily Caloric Consumption: Unknown.
Adult Obesity Rate: 10.6% (2008)
Underweight Children under Age 5: 10.6% (2004)

Gabon

Population: 1,640,286 (July 2013 est.)
Population Rank: 153rd
Population Growth Rate: 1.96% (2013 est.)
Life Expectancy at Birth: 52.15 years (2013 est.)
Health Expenditures: 3.2% of GDP (2011)
People with Access to Safe Drinking Water: 87% of population (2010 est.)
Average Daily Caloric Consumption: 2,730
Adult Obesity Rate: 13.9% (2008)
Underweight Children under Age 5: 8.8% (2001)

Republic of the Congo

Population: 4,492,689 (July 2013 est.)
Population Rank: 123rd
Population Growth Rate: 2.86% (2013 est.)
Life Expectancy at Birth: 55.6 years (2013 est.)
Health Expenditures: 2.5% of GDP (2011)
People with Access to Safe Drinking Water: 71% of population (2010 est.)
Average Daily Caloric Consumption: 2,510
Adult Obesity Rate: 4.7% (2008)
Underweight Children under Age 5: 11.8% (2005)

The countries considered here as part of Central Africa are the Democratic Republic of the Congo (DRC), the Republic of the Congo, Gabon, Equatorial Guinea, Cameroon, and the Central African Republic (CAR).

Variation in the menu is considered the key ingredient of good health. The seasonality of many foodstuffs (vegetables as well as insects) is the first step toward a balanced diet, and women will juggle the seasonal products to prepare a different dish every day. Starch dishes rarely vary; only the relish changes.

There are many food restrictions in the Central African diet, all depending on the ethnic group. Some are permanent, others only temporary. Permanent restrictions can be taboos linked to the clan. They usually concern certain types of game that are rare anyway, for example, lion, heron, or python. Sometimes the prohibition is only on the killing, and the meat in question can be consumed if killed by another person. Women are prohibited certain foods, again usually scarce meat, such as baboon and crocodile. These items are linked to strength and masculinity. A taboo can also be linked to religion. Adherents of the Kimbanguist church, a Congolese branch of Christianity, do not eat pork or monkey and do not drink alcohol. Temporary restrictions are linked to pregnancy and giving birth, to initiation, and to mourning. In the case of pregnancy the prohibition is often linked to a characteristic of the food item. Pangolin, for instance, is a mammal covered with scales that moves slowly and rolls up in a ball as a defense mechanism. The Gbaya (CAR) fear that if the parents eat pangolin, the child will have skin problems and difficulty walking. In some places women who have their periods cannot prepare food for their family. Finally, food restrictions can be used as a remedy in case of illness.

Birgit Ricquier

Further Reading

Munzele Munzimi, Jean-Macaire. *Les Pratiques de sociabilité en Afrique. Les mutations culinaires chez les Ambuun*. Paris: Publibook, 2005.

National Research Council, Board on Science and Technology for International Development. *Lost Crops of Africa*. 3 vols. Washington, DC: National Academy Press, 1996–2008.

Osseo-Asare, Fran. *Food Culture in Sub-Saharan Africa*. Westport, CT: Greenwood Press, 2005.

Côte d'Ivoire

Population: 22,400,835 (July 2013 est.)
Population Rank: 54th
Population Growth Rate: 2% (2013 est.)
Life Expectancy at Birth: 57.66 years (2013 est.)
Health Expenditures: 6.8% of GDP (2011)
People with Access to Safe Drinking Water: 80% of population (2010 est.)
Average Daily Caloric Consumption: 2,510
Adult Obesity Rate: 6.2% (2008)
Underweight Children under Age 5: 29.4% (2007)

The Côte d'Ivoire still suffers from the effects of its ongoing internal conflict. In 2006 the World Health Organization *Country Health System Fact Sheet* indicated that about 15 percent of the population was undernourished and added that 21.2 percent of the children under age five were underweight and more than 25 percent were considered short for their age, or "stunted." In March 2008 the country, along with others in western Africa, experienced food riots protesting the rising cost of staples. The country's north/south divide coupled with the urban/rural one means that rural dwellers in the northern part of the country are more subject to interrupted food supplies in the rainy seasons. The same happens in the dry season if drought occurs. The southern regions are closer to seaports and have more stable climactic conditions. The more developed economy means that there are methods of food storage, and most people can afford to purchase food from markets and other sources if their individual food supplies are destroyed.

Jessica B. Harris

Further Reading

Harris, Jessica. *The Africa Cookbook: Tastes of a Continent.* New York: Simon and Schuster, 1998.

Sheehan, Patricia, and Jacqueline Ong. *Côte d'Ivoire.* New York: Marshall Cavendish Benchmark, 2010.

Egypt

Population: 85,294,388 (July 2013 est.)
Population Rank: 15th
Population Growth Rate: 1.88% (2013 est.)
Life Expectancy at Birth: 73.19 years (2013 est.)
Health Expenditures: 4.9% of GDP (2011)
People with Access to Safe Drinking Water: 99% of population
Average Daily Caloric Consumption: 3,160
Adult Obesity Rate: 33.1% (2008)
Underweight Children under Age 5: 6.8% (2008)

The diet and health of all Egyptians cannot be easily categorized or explained. Personal tastes, lifestyles, religion, and socioeconomic factors determine what individual Egyptians eat on a daily basis. Farmers and fishermen have the healthiest diets, consisting of grains, produce, pulses, fish, and small amounts of meat. Their active lifestyles help them maintain healthy body weights, and they have low stress-related issues. Unfortunately, even though the traditional Egyptian diet is healthful and balanced, it is increasingly less popular due to working women's time constraints and the affluent's new taste preferences. Meat is the most prized item at the dinner table, and it is extremely expensive in Egypt, which deepens its image as a luxury item. Since it contains fat and cholesterol, it is not as healthy as whole grains, fruits, vegetables, and legumes. High cholesterol and heart complications are on the rise in Egypt. Four or five pounds of meat in Egypt can cost the entire week's salary of a lower-class worker. For this reason, many people joke that the poorer people are healthier. Healthful traditional whole-grain breads are increasingly being replaced by white store-bought breads, and healthful herbal and flower-based drinks are being eschewed in favor of colas. Because the culture holds a strong respect for foreign (especially American and European) products, it is widely believed that American foods are better than Egyptian ones—even if they are of poor, mass-produced quality.

Amy Riolo

T'amaya (Egyptian Fava Falafel)

Serves 4 (three falafel per person)
This recipe became popular after the fourth century CE, when Egyptian Christians (Copts) had to fast for 55 days during Lent. The Coptic fasting period prohibits meat, dairy, and seafood, so vegan diets are required. Being a meat-loving culture, the Egyptian Christians developed ingenious ways of using beans and legumes to make enticing, hearty dishes that rival their typical meaty mains.

1 c peeled dried fava beans (broad beans), soaked overnight in water and drained
$1/4$ c fresh dill leaves
$1/4$ c fresh cilantro leaves
$1/4$ c fresh parsley leaves
1 small yellow onion, diced
8 cloves garlic, chopped
1 tsp ground cumin
1 tsp ground coriander
Pinch of cayenne pepper
Salt
Freshly ground black pepper
1 tsp baking powder
Expeller-pressed corn oil, for frying
$1/4$ c white sesame seeds

Variation
4 white pita breads
2 roma tomatoes, thinly sliced

1 cucumber, thinly sliced
$1/_4$ lb feta cheese, crumbled

Place beans, dill, cilantro, parsley, onion, and garlic in a food processor and mix until a smooth paste forms. Mix in $1/_2$ cup water (or enough to make mixture wet and loose—it should resemble a thin paste). Add cumin, coriander, cayenne, and some salt and pepper to taste. Stir in baking powder and mix to incorporate. Spoon mixture into a bowl and let stand at room temperature for 1 hour.

Pour 3 inches of corn oil into a large frying pan over medium heat. When oil is hot enough to fry, a piece of bread dropped in it will turn golden and float to the top immediately. Using two teaspoons, gather a heaping teaspoonful of the paste in one spoon and carefully push it off with the other spoon, forming a round patty in the oil. Repeat the process until the pan is full—leaving a $1/_2$-inch space between the falafel. While falafel are cooking, sprinkle a few sesame seeds on the uncooked sides. Fry until falafel are dark golden brown, approximately 5 minutes; turn over, and fry the other sides until they are the same color. Line a platter with paper towels. Using a slotted spoon, lift falafel out of oil and drain on paper towels. Repeat with remaining dough.

Further Reading

Bey-Mardam, Farouk. *Ziryab: Authentic Arab Cuisine*. Woodbury, CT: Ici La Press, 2002.

Halici, Nevin. *Sufi Cuisine*. London: Saqi Books, 2005.

Segan, Francine. *The Philosopher's Kitchen: Recipes from Ancient Greece and Rome for the Modern Cook*. New York: Random House, 2004.

Zeidler, Judy. "Shavout Food: Turn Torah Fest into a Veggie Feast." *Jewish Journal of Greater Los Angeles*, June 10, 2005

Ethiopia and Eritrea

Ethiopia

Population: 93,877,025 (July 2013 est.)
Population Rank: 13th
Population Growth Rate: 2.9% (2013 est.)

Life Expectancy at Birth: 60 years (2013 est.)
Health Expenditures: 4.7% of GDP (2011)
People with Access to Safe Drinking Water: 21% of population (2010 est.)
Average Daily Caloric Consumption: 1,950
Adult Obesity Rate: 1.1% (2008)
Underweight Children under Age 5: 29.2% (2011)

Eritrea

Population: 6,233,682 (July 2013 est.)
Population Rank: 106th
Population Growth Rate: 2.36% (2013 est.)
Life Expectancy at Birth: 63.19 years (2013 est.)
Health Expenditures: 2.6% of GDP (2011)
People with Access to Safe Drinking Water: 61% of population (2008 est.)
Average Daily Caloric Consumption: 1,590
Adult Obesity Rate: 1.5% (2008)
Underweight Children under Age 5: 34.5% (2002)

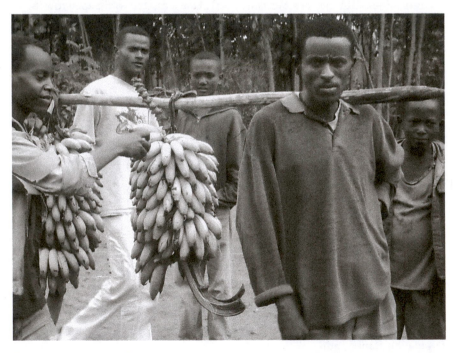

Farmers in southern Ethiopia need most of their crops to feed their families, leaving little to be sold at market for other necessities. (AP Photo/ Luc van Kemenade)

Even though the elements of the Ethiopian diet are quite nutritious, the food supply is not sufficient to meet the energy requirements of most of the population. Both man-made and environmental factors result in food insecurity. Food insecurity affects almost half the population. About 84 percent of the population is engaged in rain-fed agriculture; however, few households can produce all they need. There are few roads, and markets are not integrated, making the distribution of any surpluses across the country almost impossible.

Ethiopians do not eat much meat, eggs, or fish. Ethiopia has an abundant supply of fish, but the consumption of fish is low due to cultural taboos as well as inability to transport fish far from its original locale. Although the consumption of fruits and vegetables has increased over the past 10 years, it remains low. The per capita supply of milk and eggs has also increased but remains low.

On the positive side, 96 percent of infants begin life being breast-fed. Most infants were found to be given the breast within one hour of birth, which is a crucial statistic because some cultures believe an infant will be harmed by the mother's first milk production. Interestingly, it has been found that Ethiopian mothers with no education were more likely to practice early initiation of breast-feeding. The median duration of breast-feeding is 26 months, though there is wide variation, and the duration of breast-feeding among urban mothers is much shorter.

Another dietary deficiency is the lack of iodine, particularly in mountain regions. Vitamin A deficiency is also a problem that affects young children and mothers. Anemia is another health problem due to the low consumption of animal foods. Anemia is also compounded by endemic malaria and other parasitic diseases. The consumption of teff protects against iron deficiency because the grain is high in iron. A Food and Agriculture Organization report (United Nations, 2008) suggests that food aid to Ethiopia, which primarily consisted of wheat, actually contributed to iron deficiency because wheat, low in iron, was substituted for the traditional inclusion of teff in the diet.

Barbara J. Michael

Further Reading

Freeman, Dena. *Initiating Change in Highland Ethiopia: Causes and Consequences of Cultural Transformation.* Cambridge: Cambridge University Press, 2002.

Kifleyesus, Abbebe. "The Construction of Ethiopian National Cuisine." *Ethnorema* 3 (2006): 27–48.

Ghana

Population: 25,199,609 (July 2013 est.)
Population Rank: 48th
Population Growth Rate: 2.19% (2013 est.)
Life Expectancy at Birth: 65.32 years (2013 est.)
Health Expenditures: 4.8% of GDP (2011)
People with Access to Safe Drinking Water: 86% of population (2010 est.)
Average Daily Caloric Consumption: 2,850
Adult Obesity Rate: 7.5% (2008)
Underweight Children under Age 5: 14.3% (2008)

In 1995, the World Bank stated that 11 percent of the population was undernourished and added that 27 percent of the children under age five were underweight and more than 25 percent were considered short for their age, or "stunted." Between 1990 and 1995 one-third of all Ghanaian children had some form of goiter, which is indicative of thyroid disease. The country's north/south divide coupled with the urban/rural one meant that rural dwellers in the northern part of the country were more subject to interrupted food supplies in the rainy seasons when flooding might interrupt food sources. The same happened in the dry season if drought occurred. The southern regions are closer to seaports and have more stable climactic conditions. The more developed economy means that there are methods of food storage, and most people can afford to purchase food from markets and other sources if their individual food supplies are destroyed. The University of Ghana's Faculty of Science has a department of Nutrition and Food Science to address these issues, and the regional African office of the Food and Agriculture Organization of the United Nations is based in Accra, Ghana.

Jessica B. Harris

Further Reading

Harris, Jessica. *The Africa Cookbook: Tastes of a Continent.* New York: Simon and Schuster, 1998.

Osseo-Asare, Fran. *A Good Soup Attracts Chairs.* Baton Rouge, LA: Pelican, 1993.

Guinea

Population: 11,176,026 (July 2013 est.)
Population Rank: 75th

Population Growth Rate: 2.64% (2013 est.)
Life Expectancy at Birth: 59.11 years (2013 est.)
Health Expenditures: 6% of GDP (2011)
People with Access to Safe Drinking Water: 18% of population (2010 est.)
Average Daily Caloric Consumption: 2,530
Adult Obesity Rate: 4.4% (2008)
Underweight Children under Age 5: 20.8% (2008)

The Guinean diet is a healthy one with plenty of fresh fruit, seafood, and healthy palm oil. Minimal food processing and essentially no access to fast food have limited many diseases related to the overconsumption of highly processed, unhealthy foods. However, years of sporadic armed conflict along with governmental neglect and corruption have exacerbated poverty and accelerated the deterioration of the country's already-fragile infrastructure. Poverty has also caused ethnic tensions, while explosive population growth coupled with underdevelopment of the country's agricultural production systems has made malnutrition a real issue in Guinea, contributing to the problem of limited access to food even though a high percentage of the population works in the agricultural sector.

Overcrowding of the few hospitals and medical centers and a lack of doctors make treatment difficult even with large numbers of nongovernmental organizations running programs that target health. Only about half of all Guineans have access to clean water, and fewer than 20 percent have access to adequate sanitation. Poverty and corruption make maintaining adequate health programs a difficult task.

Rachel Finn

Further Reading

Ember, Melvin, and Carol R. Ember. "Guinea." In *Countries and Their Cultures*, 2: 942–51. New York: MacMillan Reference USA, 2001.

Osseo-Asare, Fran. *Food Culture in Sub-Saharan Africa*. Westport, CT: Greenwood Press, 2005.

Kenya

Population: 44,037,656 (July 2013 est.)
Population Rank: 31st
Population Growth Rate: 2.27% (2013 est.)
Life Expectancy at Birth: 63.29 years (2013 est.)

Health Expenditures: 4.5% of GDP (2011)
People with Access to Safe Drinking Water: 32% of population (2010 est.)
Average Daily Caloric Consumption: 2,060
Adult Obesity Rate: 4.2% (2008)
Underweight Children under Age 5: 16.4% (2009)

There are severe nutrition problems for much of the nation, made worse by the fact that 50 percent of the population is below the poverty line (2000 estimate). About 80 percent of Kenyan land gets very little rain. Less than 20 percent of the land is good for agriculture, and this 20 percent feeds 80 percent of the population. This land is overused and is being degraded. Kenya's food supply is limited, and a third of the country is undernourished. Things are getting better but only slowly. Most people get their calories each day from cereals, sugar, and vegetable oil, but the availability of fruit, vegetables, and milk is increasing.

Young children are often malnourished. Although universal breast-feeding helps greatly, it is often mixed with nonbeneficial practices such as bottle-feeding, which are made more damaging by poverty. The Food and Agriculture Organization has concluded that long-term strategies are needed such as putting additives in common food to attempt to ensure that vitamins and other micronutrients get in the diet, promoting the consumption of more diverse foods such as fruit and vegetables, and in general educating the population about good nutrition.

Robert A. Leonard

Further Reading

Holtzman, Jon. *Uncertain Tastes: Memory, Ambivalence, and the Politics of Eating in Samburu, Northern Kenya*. Berkeley: University of California Press, 2009.

Leonard, Robert. "Meaning in Nonlinguistic Systems." In *Advances in Functional Linguistics: Columbia School beyond Its Origins*, edited by Radmilla Jovanoi&#x00B4\c Gorup, Joseph Davis, and Nancy Stern, 309–34. Amsterdam, the Netherlands: John Benjamins, 2006.

Osseo-Asare, Fran. *Food Culture in Sub-Saharan Africa*. Westport, CT: Greenwood Press, 2005.

Liberia

Population: 3,989,703 (July 2013 est.)
Population Rank: 127th
Population Growth Rate: 2.56% (2013 est.)
Life Expectancy at Birth: 57.81 years (2013 est.)
Health Expenditures: 19.5% of GDP (2011)

People with Access to Safe Drinking Water: 18% of population (2010 est.)
Average Daily Caloric Consumption: 2,160
Adult Obesity Rate: 4.8% (2008)
Underweight Children under Age 5: 20.4% (2007)

Liberians eat a variety of meats, fresh fruits, and vegetables; however, the starchy staples of rice and cassava that accompany nearly every meal make the cuisine a heavy one. With civil war and unrest, the diet and health of Liberian citizens have suffered immeasurably. The civil war left the country reeling, affecting all aspects of life, particularly food production and infrastructure, which has made it even more difficult for the Liberian government to feed its citizens. As such, malnutrition is a serious issue facing the country.

Rachel Finn

Palm Butter Soup

Palm butter is a thick cream extracted from boiled, crushed palm fruits. In Liberia, people usually make it from scratch, but it is also commercially available. Palm butter soup, or palm butter stew as it is sometimes called, is a very simple dish once the palm butter has been prepared. It is a rich dish with a complex flavor that is most commonly prepared with a mix of seafood, just chicken, chicken and seafood, or chicken and beef.

2 28-oz cans palm nut cream
1 lb chicken pieces, cut small
1 c shrimp
1 c crabmeat
1 Scotch bonnet or habanero chili, finely chopped
1 medium onion, finely chopped
Salt and pepper
Fish stock (optional)

Season the chicken and shrimp with salt and pepper and set aside for 30–60 minutes. When the chicken is ready, place palm nut cream in a pot to melt. When the cream has melted, it will be rather thin. Add the chicken, onions, and chili and simmer over low heat until the chicken is done and sauce begins to thicken, about 25 minutes. Add shrimp, crabmeat, and all other ingredients and simmer 2–3 more minutes. If using fish stock, add to pot with seafood.

Further Reading

Ember, Melvin, and Carol R. Ember. "Liberia." In *Countries and Their Cultures*, 3: 1281–89. New York: MacMillan Reference USA, 2001.

Olukoju, Ayodeji. *Culture and Customs of Liberia*. Westport, CT: Greenwood Press, 2006.

Osseo-Asare, Fran. *Food Culture in Sub-Saharan Africa*. Westport, CT: Greenwood Press, 2005.

Maasai

High blood pressure, cardiac disease, and diabetes would be expected to be common among Maasai given their high-fat diet, but this is not the case as long as they continue to exercise, mostly walking long distances every day. Many Maasai succumb to disease when they give up the lifestyle of a pastoralist.

Soups are probably the most important medium for consumption of wild plant food by the Maasai. *Olkiloriti* (*Acacia nilotica*), a powerful digestive, is the most frequently used soup additive. The root or stem bark is boiled in water and the decoction drunk alone or added to soup. The Maasai are fond of taking this as a drug; it is known to make them energetic, aggressive, and fearless.

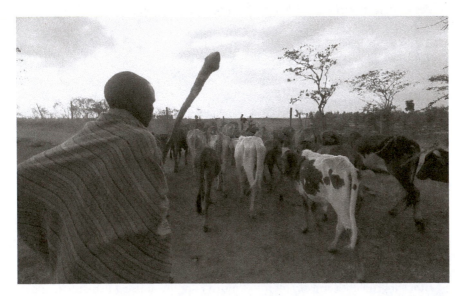

A Maasai farmer with his cattle. Recent droughts in eastern Africa have increased famine and conflict in the area. (AP Photo/Sayyid Azim)

Soups prepared during the time of a meat feast are laced with bitter bark and roots containing cholesterol-lowering saponins. Some that are added to the finishing stew on the last day of feasting have strong purgative or emetic effects.

Medicines derived from trees and shrubs are used in the treatment or prevention of a wide range of diseases and include remedies or prophylactics for malaria, sexually transmitted diseases, tuberculosis, diarrheal disorders, parasitic infestations, prostate problems, arthritis, and respiratory disorders. Particular attention is given to women's health during pregnancy and childbirth.

Kathleen Ryan

Further Reading

Homewood, K. M., P. Kristjanson, and P. Trench, eds. *Staying Maasai*. New York: Springer, 2008.

Ryan, K. "Food Sharing and Nutrition: Differential Access to Food by Age and Gender in a Pastoral Society." Paper presented at Society of Africanist Archaeologists (SAFA), Calgary, 2007.

Madagascar

Population: 22,599,098 (July 2013 est.)
Population Rank: 52nd
Population Growth Rate: 2.65% (2013 est.)
Life Expectancy at Birth: 64.85 years (2013 est.)
Health Expenditures: 4.1% of GDP (2011)
People with Access to Safe Drinking Water: 46% of population (2010 est.)
Average Daily Caloric Consumption: 2,130
Adult Obesity Rate: 1.6% (2008)
Underweight Children under Age 5: 36.8% (2004)

Madagascar has a long history of traditional medical practices (*fanafody*) that are strongly linked with the worship of ancestors. Although modern, Western hospitals and clinics are beginning to appear, they are mostly located in cities and towns, making access difficult for those living in rural areas. In addition, many Malagasy people view Western medicine, as a relatively new form of health care, with suspicion. Consequently, traditional health care is still commonplace, particularly in remote locations. Regional variations occur in methodology and treatment, but most adhere to the belief that illness is a punishment for behavior not pleasing to God—the traditionally accepted God (*Zanahary*) or the God of Christianity (*Andriamanitra*)—or the ancestors.

Traditional healers (*ombiasy*) are employed for both physical and spiritual healing, relying heavily on herbal remedies. An ombiasy is believed to have the powers of divination—connecting with the ancestors and the spirit world —to help individuals suffering from spirit possession and diagnose a variety of other illnesses. Indigenous plants and leaves are commonly used, often steeped in water as a tea or bundled and placed under the patient's bed. These herbs are believed to remedy a number of maladies including headaches, common colds, nausea, toothache, and many others. The greens (bredes) so prevalent in cooking today, for example, were first used as medicine, slowly earning a place in everyday life. Spices, roots, and animal bones are part of the ombiasy medical repertoire as well. Markets are the best place to find them; stalls overflowing with various herbal concoctions are everywhere, overseen by ombiasy eager to find patients to purchase their wares.

Rice, too, is believed to have healing properties; the soft version (sosoa) is typically served to the sick. The Malagasy believe that children are well only if they eat enough rice. Toasted, ground rice flour (lango) is considered the food of the ancestors and thought to be restorative to the health.

Perhaps the greatest threat to Malagasy health is malnourishment and the lack of potable water. As one of the poorest nations in the world, sanitation standards and access to electrical power, transportation, and running water are well below those of the West. And with 70 percent of the population living on less than one dollar a day, access to food is a serious problem. Thirty-eight percent of the population is undernourished, mostly from insufficient caloric consumption and protein deficiencies. Forty-five percent of children under the age of three have stunted growth, a result of their mothers' poor diet during pregnancy. The average life expectancy is 64 years. Cities have the best living conditions and access to plenty of food by comparison to rural areas.

Jennifer Hostetter

Romazava

Although this dish is traditionally made with beef, other meats may be substituted, including chicken or pork.

2 tbsp vegetable oil
1/2 large onion, diced
1 lb boneless beef, cut into 1-in. pieces
1 clove garlic, minced

2 tsp ginger, minced
1 chili pepper, diced
1 c canned tomatoes, diced
1 small bunch fresh spinach
1 bunch fresh watercress
1 small bunch mustard greens
Water, to cover
Salt and pepper to taste

In a large stockpot, sweat onions in oil over medium heat until translucent. Add beef and cook for approximately 10 minutes, stirring occasionally. Add garlic, ginger, and chili and cook for an additional 3 minutes. Add tomatoes and simmer for another 10 minutes. Add water and bring to a boil. Add greens and reduce heat to low. Simmer 1 hour or until meat is tender when pierced with a fork, stirring occasionally. Season with salt and pepper to taste.

Further Reading

Donenfield, Jill. *Mankafy Sakofo: Delicious Meals from Madagascar.* Lincoln, NE: iUniverse, 2007.

Jacob, Jeanne, and Michael Ashkenazi. "Madagascar." In *The World Cookbook for Students.* Vol. 3, *Iraq to Myanmar*, 128–33. Westport, CT: Greenwood Press, 2007.

Mauritania

Population: 3,437,610 (July 2013 est.)
Population Rank: 133rd
Population Growth Rate: 2.29% (2013 est.)
Life Expectancy at Birth: 61.91 years (2013 est.)
Health Expenditures: 5.4% of GDP (2011)
People with Access to Safe Drinking Water: 50% of population (2010 est.)
Average Daily Caloric Consumption: 2,820
Adult Obesity Rate: 12.7% (2008)
Underweight Children under Age 5: 15.9% (2008)

Religion influences Mauritanian dietary practices in many ways. Almost all Mauritanians are Sunni Muslims. Sunni is the largest denomination of Islam and means the words, actions, or example of the Prophet Muhammad. Mauritanians consume only halal food, which Islamic law dictates is the only food that is permissible to eat. Halal meat must be slaughtered in the way set out by Islamic law. The animal must be killed quickly, with the knife slitting the throat while a prayer is said and the name of Allah is spoken. The Quran explicitly forbids the consumption of the following foods: pork; blood; carnivorous birds of prey; animals slaughtered to anyone other than the name of Allah; carrion; an animal that has been strangled, beaten (to death), killed by a fall, gored (to death), or savaged by a beast of prey; fish that have died out of water; food over which Allah's name is not pronounced; and alcohol.

In Mauritania, the cultural ideal of beauty encourages young women to eat foods high in fat so that they gain weight. A person who is overweight by Western standards is instead considered beautiful in Mauritania. This practice is slowly diminishing as the influence of Western culture through television shows and movies takes effect.

Annie Goldberg

Further Reading

Anderson, Sarah. *Anderson's Travel Companion*. London: Pallas Athene, 2004.

Wiefels, Roland. "Mauritania: Fish Trade and Food Security in Mauritania." In *Report of the Expert Consultation on International Fish Trade and Food Security*. Rome, Italy: Food and Agriculture Organization of the United Nations, 2003.

Morocco

Population: 32,649,130 (July 2013 est.)
Population Rank: 38th
Population Growth Rate: 1.04% (2013 est.)
Life Expectancy at Birth: 76.31 years (2013 est.)
Health Expenditures: 6% of GDP (2011)
People with Access to Safe Drinking Water: 83% of population (2010 est.)
Average Daily Caloric Consumption: 3,230
Adult Obesity Rate: 16.4% (2008)
Underweight Children under Age 5: 3.1% (2011)

Moroccans consume a Mediterranean diet featuring many fruits and vegetables. Fish is a major food in coastal regions, and garlic and olive oil figure in many dishes. The oil of the indigenous argan tree is high in unsaturated fats. However, it is laborious to produce and too expensive for most Moroccans.

On the whole, the Moroccan diet is rather high in carbohydrates, and in recent decades there has been a growing but not well-understood problem of obesity in urban areas, particularly among women, 18 percent of whom are now obese, as opposed to 5.7 percent of men. This is rate is more than triple what it was in 1980, when male and female obesity were roughly equal. The traditional dietary problem had been malnutrition, which still exists to some extent, particularly among children in rural areas.

A more serious problem in rural regions is availability of safe drinking water. In the countryside, only 58 percent of people have access to safe water, and many people suffer from gastrointestinal infections. In the cities, 100 percent of the water is considered safe.

Charles Perry

Qotban (Brochettes)

Serves 8–10 as a snack or appetizer
Qotban (literally, "sticks") are typically made by marinating the meat with vinegar, onions, and pepper. This version from the Atlantic coast is more elaborately flavored, giving an idea of the variety of spices used in Morocco.

3 lb leg of lamb
2$^1/_2$ tsp cumin
2 tsp paprika
1$^1/_2$ tsp white pepper
1 tsp black pepper
1 tsp turmeric
1 tsp oregano
3 bay leaves, crumbled
$^1/_2$ onion, minced
3 cloves garlic, minced
$^1/_4$ c olive oil
1 tbsp red wine vinegar
2 oz ($^1/_2$ stick) butter, melted
1 tbsp cumin

Cut the lamb into about 15 (¾-inch) cubes. In a mixing bowl, mix the cumin, paprika, white pepper, black pepper, turmeric, oregano, and bay leaves. Add the meat and rub with the spices. Toss with the onion, garlic, oil, and vinegar. Cover and refrigerate 24 hours.

Arrange the chunks of meat on skewers and grill until done to taste, about 7–8 minutes, basting with melted butter every 5 minutes. Dust with cumin and serve.

Further Reading

Heine, Peter. *Food Culture in the Middle East and North Africa.* Westport, CT: Greenwood Press, 2004.

Peterson, Joan. *Eat Smart in Morocco: How to Decipher the Menu, Know the Market Foods and Embark on a Tasting Adventure.* Berkeley, CA: Ginkgo Press, 2002.

Mozambique

Population: 24,096,669 (July 2013 est.)

Population Rank: 50th

Population Growth Rate: 2.44% (2013 est.)

Life Expectancy at Birth: 52.29 years (2013 est.)

Health Expenditures: 6.6% of GDP (2011)

People with Access to Safe Drinking Water: 47% of population (2010 est.)

Average Daily Caloric Consumption: 2,070

Adult Obesity Rate: 4.9% (2008)

Underweight Children under Age 5: 18.3% (2008)

In 1975, when Mozambique gained its independence, the government created a free, nationalized health care system. Its goal was to improve the population's health through preventive medicine. They employed nurses to give

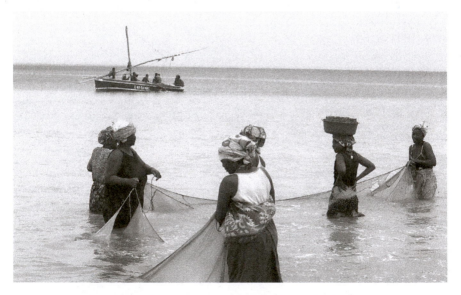

Women in Mozambique fish with nets. (Andrea Basile/Dreamstime.com)

vaccinations and to educate the population about sanitation and other basic health care issues. They established clinics throughout the country, many of which unfortunately were destroyed during the civil war. In 1992, when the civil war ended, the government began rebuilding those clinics. The government also abandoned a law prohibiting private practice in an effort to increase the number of doctors, whose numbers had dwindled due to the exodus at the beginning of the civil war. Today, the main health threats are malaria, AIDS, and sleeping sickness, which is transmitted by the tsetse fly.

Malnutrition is also a concern and is the most common health problem, mainly because there is a lack of a variety of foods in many residents' diets, and they do not consume an adequate amount of protein, vitamins, and other essential minerals. There is a movement for the population to introduce new crops and change their diet to a much healthier one. As a result, vegetable gardens are being encouraged, and beans, tomatoes, onions, potatoes, and cabbage are being planted. Many people would have to borrow money to buy the seeds to plant these crops because most Mozambicans do not have a bank account. Bananas and cashews grow well in most parts of the country and are part of the local diet. Goats are kept by many, and therefore goat milk is available. For those living along the coast and near rivers, fish and other seafood are an important part of their diet. Corn, which is often ground into flour, is eaten by people in the rural areas for most of their meals. Rice is not grown in the northern region, which means that villagers have to purchase it. Many cannot afford to do so.

Cherie Y. Hamilton

Further Reading

Hamilton, Cherie Y. *Cuisines of Portuguese Encounters*. New York: Hippocrene Books, 2008.

Rowan, Marielle. *Flavors of Mozambique*. Maputo, Mozambique: Edição do autor, 1998.

Namibia

Population: 2,182,852 (July 2013 est.)
Population Rank: 142nd
Population Growth Rate: 0.75% (2013 est.)
Life Expectancy at Birth: 52.03 years (2013 est.)
Health Expenditures: 5.3% of GDP (2011)
People with Access to Safe Drinking Water: 32% of population (2010 est.)

Average Daily Caloric Consumption: 2,350
Adult Obesity Rate: 9.5% (2008)
Underweight Children under Age 5: 17.5% (2007)

While urbanization has meant exposure to processed foods, supermarkets, and chain eateries for many Namibians, the majority of the country lives and eats in rural villages and towns where their diet has remained relatively unchanged for generations. Namibia has one of the widest gaps between rich and poor in the world, which affects diet and health indicators. While life expectancy in Namibia is an average of 52 years, if calculated along class and race lines, a more divergent set of ages would be revealed.

Anita Verna Crofts

Further Reading

Anandajayasekeram, Ponniah, Mandivamba Rukani, Suresh Babu, and Frikkie Liebenberg, eds. *Impact of Science on African Agriculture and Food Security.* Wallingford, UK: CABI, 2007.

Chavonnes Vrugt, Antoinette de. *My Hungry Heart: Notes from a Namibian Kitchen.* Birmingham, AL: Venture, 2009.

Nigeria

Population: 174,507,539 (July 2013 est.)
Population Rank: 7th
Population Growth Rate: 2.54% (2013 est.)
Life Expectancy at Birth: 52.46 years (2013 est.)
Health Expenditures: 5.3% of GDP (2011)
People with Access to Safe Drinking Water: 58% of population (2010 est.)
Average Daily Caloric Consumption: 2,710
Adult Obesity Rate: 6.5% (2008)
Underweight Children under Age 5: 26.7% (2008)

Given the relative productivity of the land and the possibility of growing a large variety of fruits and vegetables, the country offers the potential for providing access to a good, well-rounded diet. Indeed, recent estimates suggest that the average Nigerian's daily calorie supply is around 2,700. However, the extreme poverty of so many can be linked to health inequalities that are directly related to or are impacted on by diet. Of children under the age of five, about 39 percent are underweight, and over 39 percent are stunted (short for their age). Just over one-quarter of all children under five (27%) are estimated to be malnourished. Many in Nigeria also suffer from vitamin A deficiencies, which can result in blindness; these deficiencies result from inadequate access to greens, orange fruits and vegetables, and protein. As is the case with food supplies, access to clean drinking water is also divided by class. Just 51 percent of the population has access to safe drinking water, while the remainder are susceptible to waterborne diseases such as bacterial and protozoal diarrhea, hepatitis A and E, and typhoid fever. Nigeria is also in a malarial zone. These diseases can also contribute to vitamin A deficiency.

Finally, while malnutrition and water-related illness certainly contribute to the short life expectancy, AIDS also takes its toll. Today, the estimated life expectancy of Nigerian men and women is 52 years. Nearly 3 million adults in Nigeria are living with AIDS or HIV. Antiretrovirals, which are used to treat AIDS, are costly and require doctor support; also, the person must take the drugs with food and must take them several times a day. Access to food and water plays an intrinsic role in the life chances of Nigerians today, because without access the cycle of poverty is further exacerbated.

Intergenerational transfer of illnesses such as AIDS and illnesses related to vitamin and mineral deficiencies such as goiter, night blindness, and rickets are also linked to poverty. The estimated infant mortality rate was over 7 percent, or about 74 infant deaths for every 1,000 live births. Importantly, newborns in Nigerian societies are regarded with pride. They represent a community's and a family's future and often are the main reason for many marriages (a large proportion of Nigerian households are characterized by polygamy). Throughout Nigeria, the bond between mother and child is very strong. During the first few years of a child's life, the mother is never far away, and Nigerian women place great importance on breast-feeding and the bond that it creates between mother and child. Children are often not weaned off their mother's milk until they are toddlers. If a mother is infected with AIDS or HIV or is vitamin deficient herself, then her milk will not be sufficient to adequately feed her child.

Both Western and traditional forms of medicine are available in Nigeria. The health care system is sponsored by the government; however, because corruption is high and there is a shortage of trained health care professionals, ordinary Nigerians' access to health care is limited. Traditional medicine, also known as *juju*, is commonly practiced and involves the use of a variety of plants and herbs in the cures. Most families also have their own secret remedies for minor health problems. Juju can also involve adhering to food taboos; for example, when suffering from breathing difficulties one should avoid hot food, kola nuts, and coconuts. Likewise, "slimy" food (e.g., okra soup) should be avoided when recovering from a wound because it is thought that the wound needs to dry out to heal and the texture of the foods will slow this process down. Some traditional remedies involve avoiding foods that, while not related to the characteristics of the malady, when eaten are thought to anger the gods. For example, smallpox is thought to worsen if chicken and grains are consumed because for some these foods are forbidden and the gods will not heal the patient if they are eaten. Finally, the character of the overall diet is also linked to understandings that combine taste with health benefits. Pepper, for instance, is used not just to improve the flavor of the dish but also because it is thought to act as a natural preservative and antibacterial agent and also to reduce the body temperature of the eater, which is important in a hot climate.

Megan K. Blake

Groundnut Stew

Serves 6

1 stewing chicken or chicken parts (2–3 lb)
2–3 tsp oil for frying
1 tsp salt
A pinch of cayenne pepper
1 yellow onion, chopped finely
1–2 garlic cloves, chopped
4 c water
1 1/2 c natural peanut butter (preferably with low sugar content)
Cooked rice for 6
Toppings: Chopped tomato, onions, pineapple, orange, papaya, banana, and grated coconut

In a large heavy-bottomed pan, heat the oil and fry the onion and garlic until soft (5–10 minutes). Add the cayenne pepper. Once the onions and garlic start to caramelize, add the chicken and cover with water to form a broth. Simmer until tender. Once the chicken is cooked, remove the chicken from the broth and debone. Add the peanut butter to the cooking broth and stir until smooth. Return the deboned chicken to the broth and simmer for a half hour or more. If a thicker sauce is desired, it can be thickened with cornstarch. Adjust seasoning to taste. Serve over cooked rice (as you would a curry) and sprinkle with fruit toppings.

Further Reading

Falola, Toyin. *Culture and Customs of Nigeria*. Westport, CT: Greenwood Press, 2000.

Gordon, April A. *Nigeria's Diverse Peoples: A Reference Sourcebook*. Santa Barbara, CA: ABC-CLIO, 2003.

Robson, E. "The 'Kitchen' as Women's Space in Rural Hausaland, Northern Nigeria." *Gender, Place and Culture* 13, No. 6 (2006): 669–76.

Senegal

Population: 13,300,410 (July 2013 est.)
Population Rank: 71st
Population Growth Rate: 2.51% (2013 est.)
Life Expectancy at Birth: 60.57 years (2013 est.)
Health Expenditures: 6% of GDP (2011)
People with Access to Safe Drinking Water: 52% of population (2010 est.)
Average Daily Caloric Consumption: 2,320
Adult Obesity Rate: 6.8% (2008)
Underweight Children under Age 5: 19.2% (2011)

Malnutrition has historically been and continues to be a serious concern in Senegal. In turn, calorie-dense foods like oil and meat are highly valued, because they are believed to give strength and to symbolize wealth. Until recently, in many parts of Senegal, it was said that when eating a good ceebu jën, one should have oil running down one's arm. The energy-filled carbohydrate bases of meals vary little, whereas the quantity of vegetables, fish, and meat lessens significantly in times of economic downturn.

Foods that are very sweet, salty, and oily are highly appreciated in Senegal, perhaps in part related to the constant threat of malnutrition. But diet-related noncommunicable diseases are increasingly widespread and are transforming ideas concerning health and nutrition. Diabetes and cardiac disease are extremely prevalent in Senegal and are a significant cause of death in the country. These degenerative diseases have been the subjects of many public awareness campaigns. Senegalese are thus increasingly familiar with problems related to obesity and consuming too much fat, cholesterol, and sugar.

However, awareness does not necessarily equate to transformations in eating habits. Senegalese often lament that their food is excessively oily, salty, or sweet but often feel that it is unalterable. This is, in part, due to the social role of eating in Senegalese society. Meals are a time of social exchange. Families eat together and welcome guests; meals link social networks. If one person or one family drastically changed their eating habits, this could isolate them and would seem individualistic and selfish.

The social difficulties of changing one's eating habits for health are obvious in the experiences of diabetics. Diabetics often explain that it is extremely difficult to avoid drinking sugary beverages because these play a critical role in welcoming a guest. To turn down food or drink one has been offered is considered discourteous. Familial celebrations pose a similar problem. To avoid appearing rude or ungrateful, diabetics often hide their illness and eat the foods offered, regardless of their nutritional content.

The price of ingredients and the cultural perception of ideal body size also play important roles in nutritional choices. It is cheaper to feed a large family a diet based on rice and oil than one based on vegetables. Many Senegalese simply do not have the economic means to consume the daily recommended amount of fruits and vegetables. In addition, heaviness is often associated with wealth, motherliness, and health. In turn, Senegalese women often prefer body sizes that are considered overweight by Western medical standards and make dietary choices based on these cultural perceptions rather than health considerations.

Despite the many cultural obstacles that inhibit proper nutrition, more and more Senegalese are attempting to make healthful changes in their diets. Many are trying to incorporate more fruits and vegetables into their diets and to avoid consuming excess rice, oil, salt, and sugar. These changes are mainly taking place in middle- and upper-class families, whose economic means allow them a certain nutritional flexibility that lower classes do not have.

Chelsie Yount

Further Reading

N'Dour, Youssou. *Sénégal: La cuisine de ma mère*. Geneva, Switzerland: Éditions Minerva, 2004.

Osseo-Asare, Fran. *Food Culture in Sub-Saharan Africa*. Westport, CT: Greenwood Press, 2005.

Sierra Leone

Population: 5,612,685 (July 2013 est.)
Population Rank: 110th
Population Growth Rate: 2.3% (2013 est.)
Life Expectancy at Birth: 56.98 years (2013 est.)
Health Expenditures: 18.8% of GDP (2011)
People with Access to Safe Drinking Water: 13% of population (2010 est.)
Average Daily Caloric Consumption: 2,130
Adult Obesity Rate: 6.8% (2008)
Underweight Children under Age 5: 21.3% (2008)

Sierra Leoneans have a varied diet that includes seafood, meat, many fresh fruits and vegetables, and very limited amounts of processed or sugary foods. Even with high amounts of rice and palm oil in their diets, most health problems do not stem from the typical diet itself. Rather, lack of food and subsequent malnutrition and inadequate sanitation are the primary causes of health problems in Sierra Leone. Civil war and governmental abuses have caused crushing poverty and a crumbling infrastructure. Basic food production and health care systems have been neglected, making it impossible to meet the needs of the growing population. While things are stabilizing slowly, hunger and malnutrition continue to be issues facing the people and government of Sierra Leone.

Rachel Finn

Further Reading

Ember, Melvin, and Carol R. Ember. "Sierra Leone." In *Countries and Their Cultures*, 1982–93. New York: MacMillan Reference USA, 2001.

Osseo-Asare, Fran. *Food Culture in Sub-Saharan Africa*. Westport, CT: Greenwood Press, 2005.

Somalia

Population: 10,251,568 (July 2013 est.)
Population Rank: 84th
Population Growth Rate: 1.67% (2013 est.)
Life Expectancy at Birth: 51.19 years (2013 est.)

Health Expenditures: Unknown
People with Access to Safe Drinking Water: 29% of population (2010 est.)
Average Daily Caloric Consumption: Unknown
Adult Obesity Rate: 4.8% (2008)
Underweight Children under Age 5: 32.8% (2006)

Religion influences Somali dietary practices in a number of ways. Nearly all Somalis are Sunni Muslims. Sunni is the largest denomination of Islam and means the words, actions, or example of the Prophet Muhammad. Muslim Somalis consume only halal food, which Islamic law dictates is the only food that is permissible to eat. Halal meat must be slaughtered in the way set out by Islamic law. The animal must be killed quickly, with the knife slitting the throat while a prayer is said and the name of Allah is spoken. The Quran explicitly forbids the consumption of the following foods: pork; blood; carnivorous birds of prey; animals slaughtered to anyone other than the name of Allah; carrion; an animal that has been strangled, beaten (to death), killed by a fall, gored (to death), or savaged by a beast of prey; fish that have died out of water; food over which Allah's name is not pronounced; and alcohol.

Annie Goldberg

Canjeero

This bread is a staple in the Somali diet. It can be eaten with every meal. Traditionally, it is made with corn or sorghum flour.

2 c sorghum or corn flour
2 2/3 c lukewarm water

Whisk together the flour and water until a smooth batter forms. Let the batter rest.

Grease a nonstick or cast iron pan with ghee and heat over medium low. Pour the batter into the center of the pan and rotate the pan so that the batter evenly coats the bottom. Cook until the batter has set and is no longer sticky. Do not flip the bread to cook on the other side. Simply remove it from the pan and serve it as an accompaniment to a meal or plain with sugar and ghee.

Further Reading

Ali, Barlin. *Somali Cuisine*. Bloomington, IN: Author House, 2007.

Anderson, Sarah. *Sarah Anderson's Travel Companion: Africa and the Middle East*. London: Pallas Athene, 2004.

South Africa

Population: 48,601,098 (July 2013 est.)
Population Rank: 26th
Population Growth Rate: –0.45% (2013 est.)
Life Expectancy at Birth: 49.48 years (2013 est.)
Health Expenditures: 8.5% of GDP (2011)
People with Access to Safe Drinking Water: 91% of population (2010 est.)
Average Daily Caloric Consumption: 2,950
Adult Obesity Rate: 31.3% (2008)
Underweight Children under Age 5: 11.6% (2005)

Echoing all other spheres of South African life, people with financial means can benefit from first-rate private health care, while the majority of South Africans currently have access only to the very rudimentary health care that the government provides free of charge. One result of this is an average life expectancy of 49 years, concentrated in the 80 percent majority who do not have access to adequate health services.

HIV is the biggest health challenge that South Africa faces, with a prevalence of close to 20 percent and over 5 million people living with the virus. It has also been the subject of the most notorious link between diet and health, when, in the period 2000–2005, then-president Thabo Mbeki denied the causal relationship between HIV and AIDS and publicly recommended eating a diet rich in fruit and vegetables to fight the disease, rather than prioritizing access to antiretroviral drugs. It is estimated that 350,000 people died unnecessarily during that time.

As cattle are a symbol of wealth, excess body weight is also traditionally regarded as a sign of prosperity. This continues in many black communities and is exacerbated by high rates of HIV and AIDS, now commonly considered a "slim disease" because of its associated weight loss. But the principle that being fat is healthy is also complicated by escalating rates of diabetes and related health complications resulting from overweight and obesity. While increasingly Western lifestyles in urban areas, involving higher

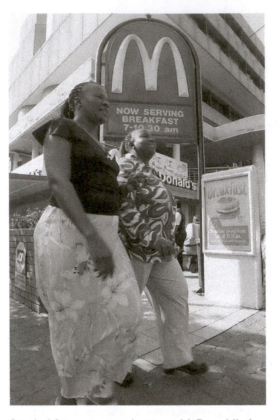

South African women leaving a McDonald's fast food restaurant near Pretoria. (AP Photo/Obed Zilwa)

consumption of fast food and convenience foods, have contributed to this development, it is also the result of traditional ways of life across most racial groups, as eating substantial portions of meat and starch, often coupled with large amounts of beer, is not confined to black communities (white men count among the most obese in the country).

In cities the opposite trend is widespread, with a visible increase in the number of gyms, many of which work in partnership with medical insurance companies to offer reduced membership rates. Also on the rise are healthy fast-food options, from chains like Kauai (which also operate in the ubiquitous Virgin Active gyms) and Osumo, both of which specialize in smoothies, salads, sandwiches, and wraps and offer nutritional information with their menus. Leading supermarkets also have health sections that offer a number of "lite" and "low-carb" snack and meal-replacement products under leading diet brands like Weigh-Less, as well as a full array of gluten- and sugar-free foods.

Signe Rousseau

Further Reading

Leipoldt, Louis. *Leipoldt's Food and Wine*. Cape Town, South Africa: Stonewall, 2004.

Snyman, Lannice. *Rainbow Cuisine*. Cologne, Germany: Könemann, 2001.

Sudan

Population: 34,847,910 (July 2013 est.)
Population Rank: 35th
Population Growth Rate: 1.83% (2013 est.)
Life Expectancy at Birth: 62.95 years (2013 est.)
Health Expenditures: 8.4% of GDP (2011)
People with Access to Safe Drinking Water: 58% of population (2010 est.)
Average Daily Caloric Consumption: 2,270
Adult Obesity Rate: 6% (2008)
Underweight Children under Age 5: 31.7% (2006)

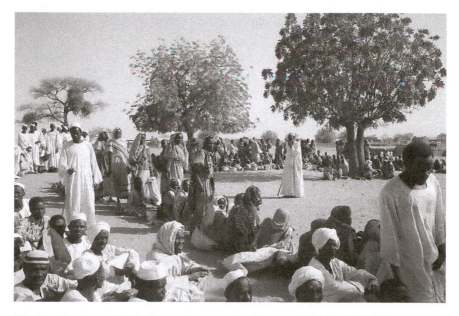

Displaced persons in Darfur wait to receive international food aid. The war in Darfur killed tens of thousands, many as the result of famine. (USAID)

While the introduction of fast food and large supermarkets in the urban areas has meant a shift in diet for some Sudanese, most Sudanese still live in small villages and towns, and their diet remains largely the same as that of their ancestors. As Sudan continues to urbanize, this trend will shift accordingly. The life expectancy in Sudan is an average of almost 63 years, not as a result of diet but instead because of a continuous cycle of food scarcity, war, diminished health facilities, and disease.

Anita Verna Crofts

Further Reading

Bacon, Josephine, and Jenni Fleetwood. *The Complete Illustrated Food and Cooking of Africa and the Middle East: Ingredients, Techniques, 170 Recipes, 650 Photographs*. London: Lorenz Books, 2009.

Grant, Rosamund, and Josephine Bacon. *The Taste of Africa: The Undiscovered Food and Cooking of an Extraordinary Continent*. London: Southwater, 2008.

Swaziland

Population: 1,403,362 (July 2013 est.)
Population Rank: 154th
Population Growth Rate: 1.17% (2013 est.)
Life Expectancy at Birth: 50.01 years (2013 est.)
Health Expenditures: 8% of GDP (2011)
People with Access to Safe Drinking Water: 71% of population (2010 est.)
Average Daily Caloric Consumption: 2,310
Adult Obesity Rate: 19.7% (2008)
Underweight Children under Age 5: 6.1% (2007)

Food restrictions in the Swazi diet are adhered to but not as commonly as before. Within the culture there is a strong awareness of the relationship between food, health, and body fat. Weight is a sign of prosperity. An underweight or thin person is a sign of poor diet. Milk is seen as an important beverage. It is drunk daily and seen as purifying during ritual occasions. While women are allowed to drink milk throughout most times in their lives, they are restricted from, or have limited contact with, the cows themselves. Depending on the woman's stage of life, contact between her and cattle is believed to affect the breeding and milk production of the cow.

Food restrictions were common. For example, adults who were still able to bear children were not to eat the meat of an aborted animal because it was believed that if they became pregnant they would have a miscarriage. Only the elderly were allowed to eat liver because, if younger people consumed it, it was thought that they would become forgetful. Men and older adults were not to eat soft porridge because it would cause them to become weak and lazy. Sugarcane and groundnuts were not to be consumed by pregnant women because of the belief that these would affect the baby once it was born. Sugarcane is said to cause a mucus-covered baby once it is born. Groundnuts are thought to cause the mother to give birth to a dirty baby. Some of the older generations still abide by these rules; however, the younger generations do not follow many food restrictions, as they cannot remember them.

Since the new millennium, food prices have been on the rise, making it difficult for the average Swazi family, especially when taking into account the prevalence of HIV/AIDS in the society. Many of those infected with the disease require well-balanced diets to facilitate the effectiveness of their antiretroviral treatments. With the increase in food prices it is difficult for these families to obtain the proper foodstuffs.

Kristina Lupp

Impala (African Antelope)

Serves 12

1 impala leg (venison may be substituted)
4 cloves garlic, sliced thinly
1 c green olives, halved
Cooking oil
3 large potatoes, diced
3 large carrots, diced
4 onions, diced
1 c beef broth
10 dried prunes, pitted
Salt and pepper to taste

Rinse the meat and pat dry.

Remove the lower shank bone and set leg aside. Place the lower shank bone into a pot, and add water to cover. Set to simmer until reduced by half.

With a sharp paring knife cut slits throughout the leg. Into the slits place the garlic and olives. Season the leg with salt and pepper.

Place the leg into a roasting pan lightly coated with oil and cook at 325°F for 25 minutes per pound.

When done, remove the leg from the pan and set aside to rest.

Meanwhile, sauté the vegetables in cooking oil until they are soft and translucent but not browned. Add the prunes and cook until soft. Strain and set the vegetables aside.

Add the broth to the juices remaining in the pan and reduce by half. To serve, place the leg on a dish with the vegetables and prunes surrounding it, and drizzle the gravy over the top.

Further Reading

Kgaphola, Mmantoa S., and Annemarie T. Viljoen. "Food Habits of Rural Swazi Households: 1939–1999, Part 1: Technological Influences on Swazi Food Habits." *Tydskrit vir Gesinsekologie en Verbruikerswetenskappe* 28 (2000): 68–74.

Kgaphola, Mmantoa S., and Annemarie T. Viljoen. "Food Habits of Rural Swazi Households: 1939–1999, Part 2: Social Structural and Ideological influences on Swazi Food Habits." *Journal of Family Ecology and Consumer Sciences* 32 (2004): 16–25.

Osseo-Asare, Fran. *Food Culture in Sub-Saharan Africa.* Westport, CT: Greenwood Press, 2005.

Uganda

Population: 34,758,809 (July 2013 est.)
Population Rank: 36th
Population Growth Rate: 3.32% (2013 est.)
Life Expectancy at Birth: 53.98 years (2013 est.)
Health Expenditures: 9.5% of GDP (2011)
People with Access to Safe Drinking Water: 72% of population (2010 est.)
Average Daily Caloric Consumption: 2,250
Adult Obesity Rate: 4.3% (2008)
Underweight Children under Age 5: 16.4% (2006)

While many Ugandan adults over the age of 45 take health into consideration and have given up meat and fried foods, and instead resort to boiled food and low-sodium dishes, the young continue to eat both traditional foods and a wide array of Western junk foods high in fat, sodium, and refined sugar.

Ken Albala and Roger Serunyigo

Further Reading

Henson, Erica. *The Food Holiday Uganda*. Atlanta: Echo Media, 2010.

Uganda: Growing Out of Poverty. Washington, DC: World Bank, 1993

Zimbabwe

Population: 13,182,908 (July 2013 est.)

Population Rank: 72nd

Population Growth Rate: 4.38% (2013 est.)

Life Expectancy at Birth: 53.86 years (2013 est.)

Health Expenditures: Unknown

People with Access to Safe Drinking Water: 40% of population (2010 est.)

Average Daily Caloric Consumption: 2,210

Adult Obesity Rate: 7% (2008)

Underweight Children under Age 5: 10.1% (2011)

The traditional rural diet is nutritionally sound in that it has few fats, uses natural rather than processed sugar, and incorporates many of the fruits that are able to grow in the country. Indeed, in the not-so-distant past, Zimbabwe was a net exporter of food. This diet has sometimes been impacted significantly by drought and crop failure, but the structural adjustment policies of the 1990s, and the more recent economic and agricultural mismanagement, have meant that this is a country plagued by an inadequate food supply. Lack of food contributes to a host of health problems that subsequently arise from starvation and malnutrition, such as blindness as a result of vitamin A deficiency and goiter due to lack of iodine in the diet. Children are stricken with kwashiorkor, a form of malnutrition linked to a lack of protein in the diet. Kwashiorkor usually affects children under five and exhibits symptoms such as a swollen belly or swollen ankles. Adults are more likely to exhibit pellagra, identified by dermatitis, diarrhea, and distemper, which is caused by niacin deficiency resulting from a diet solely of corn. Nearly two out of every five people are considered undernourished, and nearly one in every six children under age five is underweight, while one in five is stunted.

The life expectancy in Zimbabwe was identified as the lowest in the world in 2006. At that time, men are expected to live to the age of 37 and women to the age of 34. A 2013 estimate, however, has placed life expectancy at almost 54 years. The infant mortality rate is also high, at 13.5 percent; about one in every eight children dies before reaching age five. Much of the decline in health is due to the prevalence of AIDS and HIV. Approximately one-fifth of those age 20–49 are currently infected with HIV. Additionally, the low life expectancy coupled with the economic disadvantages of women (employment is concentrated in the informal and illegal trading sector, and women are responsible for paying for their children's food) means that poverty is disproportionately borne by children. Just over a third of the country's total population is composed of children under the age of 14, a large proportion of whom are orphans. Estimates in 2007 were 1.3 million orphans as a result of AIDS. They must fend for themselves or rely on an ever-shrinking pool of elderly relatives.

Unlike its neighbors, until recently Zimbabwe has had relatively safe drinking water. However, in 2008, large areas of the country were struck by cholera, which infected over 10,000 people. Typhoid fever, malaria, and schistosomiasis (a parasite-derived disease) are also present throughout the country, with those in rural areas more susceptible, as only 37 percent of those in rural areas have access to sanitation, compared with 63 percent of those in urban areas. Generally, access to water is increasingly under stress as a result of more frequent droughts brought on by global warming.

In Zimbabwe, the health system has largely failed. By the end of 2008, only one of the four major hospitals within the country was still open, and the medical school had closed. As a result, many turn to traditional healers for medical help. Traditional medicine is holistic and is concerned with healing the root cause of an illness rather than just the symptoms. The illness may be the result of having angered the ancestors by failing to follow socioreligious obligations and taboos such as those against elder abuse and promiscuity. Diet and herbs are important for curing these unnatural diseases. For example, among the Ndebele, eating food that shares one's name is prohibited. For instance, if a man's last name is "cow," then he should avoid all beef.

Megan K. Blake

Dovi (Peanut Butter Stew)

Serves 6

Oil or butter for frying
2 medium onions, chopped finely
Garlic, crushed
1 tsp salt
$1/2$ tsp pepper

$^1/_2$ tsp cayenne pepper

2 green peppers, chopped

Chicken pieces (optional)

3–4 tomatoes

2 c water

6 tbsp peanut butter

1 large bag spinach or some other green leafy vegetable or okra

In a large heavy-bottomed pot, brown the onions over medium heat in the oil or butter. When the onions are just brown, add the garlic, salt, pepper, and cayenne, and cook for a further 3–4 minutes, stirring. Add the chopped peppers and chicken, if using. Cook for about 5 minutes or until the chicken is browned. Add the tomatoes and the water, and simmer for 10 minutes. Add the peanut butter, and continue to simmer for 5 minutes. Add the spinach or other greens, and cook briefly until the leaves are limp and tender. Serve immediately.

Further Reading

Arnold, J. R., and R. W. Lener. *Robert Mugabe's Zimbabwe*. Minneapolis, MN: 21st Century Books, 2008.

Chataway, N. *The Bulawayo Cookery Book*. London: Jeppestown, 1909.

Middle East

Arabian Peninsula

Bahrain

Population: 1,281,332 July 2013 est.
Population Rank: 156th
Population Growth Rate: 2.57% (2013 est.)
Life Expectancy at Birth: 78.43 years (2013 est.)
Health Expenditures: 3.8% of GDP (2011)
People with Access to Safe Drinking Water: 100% of population (2010 est.)
Average Daily Caloric Consumption: Unknown
Adult Obesity Rate: 32.9% (2008)
Underweight Children under Age 5: Unknown or Negligible

Kuwait

Population: 2,695,316 (July 2013 est.)
Population Rank: 140th
Population Growth Rate: 1.79% (2013 est.)
Life Expectancy at Birth: 77.46 years (2013 est.)
Health Expenditures: 2.7% of GDP (2011)
People with Access to Safe Drinking Water: 99% of population (2010 est.)
Average Daily Caloric Consumption: 3,040
Adult Obesity Rate: 42% (2008)
Underweight Children under Age 5: 1.7% (2009)

Qatar

Population: 2,042,444 (July 2013 est.)
Population Rank: 146th
Population Growth Rate: 4.19% (2013 est.)
Life Expectancy at Birth: 78.24 years (2013 est.)
Health Expenditures: 1.9% of GDP (2011)
People with Access to Safe Drinking Water: 100% of population (2010 est.)

Average Daily Caloric Consumption: Unknown
Adult Obesity Rate: 33.2% (2008)
Underweight Children under Age 5: Unknown or Negligible

Saudi Arabia

Population: 26,939,583 (July 2013 est.)
Population Rank: 46th
Population Growth Rate: 1.51% (2013 est.)
Life Expectancy at Birth: 74.58 years (2013 est.)
Health Expenditures: 3.7% of GDP (2011)
People with Access to Safe Drinking Water: 97% of population (2010 est.)
Average Daily Caloric Consumption: 3,130
Adult Obesity Rate: 33% (2008)
Underweight Children under Age 5: 5.3% (2005)

United Arab Emirates (UAE)

Population: 5,473,972 (July 2013 est.)
Population Rank: 114th
Population Growth Rate: 2.87% (2013 est.)
Life Expectancy at Birth: 76.91 years (2013 est.)
Health Expenditures: 3.3% of GDP (2011)
People with Access to Safe Drinking Water: 100% of population (2010 est.)
Average Daily Caloric Consumption: 3,140
Adult Obesity Rate: 32.7% (2008)
Underweight Children under Age 5: Unknown or Negligible

The Arabian Peninsula encompasses Bahrain, Kuwait, Qatar, Saudi Arabia, and the United Arab Emirates (UAE).

The basic diet of the Arabian Peninsula is a healthy one, relatively like the modern Mediterranean food pyramid, featuring meat in moderation and an emphasis on fruit, vegetables, and grains. However, the area has developed an epidemic of obesity and related health problems. Causative factors include the social nature of eating, leading to long stays around the table; the relative abundance of food in the area since World War II; the extremely hot climate, which discourages outdoor exercise; and the prevalence of televisions and computers, encouraging a sedentary lifestyle.

Before the advent of the oil companies, for the most part Arabs depended on traditional medicine, which made use of herbs, spices, and other natural

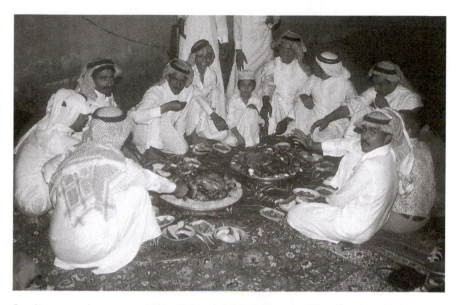

Saudi men gather around a traditional Arabian dinner. (Corel)

ingredients. Some of these items were local plants; others are spices from India, China, and other remote parts of the world. Even petroleum, which was found in seeps in some areas, was used for medicinal purposes, both as a salve and taken by mouth. Even today, petroleum jelly is an ingredient in ointments and cosmetics.

Since the discovery of oil, the availability of modern medical care has increased greatly, with hospitals providing all the medical services found in the West, including organ transplants. In Saudi Arabia, the average life expectancy at birth in 1975 was 54 years, when good medical care was already available, and it has risen to the mid-70s. Other countries on the peninsula have similar numbers.

Christine Crawford-Oppenheimer

Further Reading

Al-Hamad, Sarah. *Cardamom and Lime: Recipes from the Arabian Gulf.* Northampton, MA: Interlink, 2008.

Bsisu, May S. *The Arab Table: Recipes and Culinary Traditions.* New York: HarperCollins, 2005.

Heine, Peter. *Food Culture in the Near East, Middle East, and North Africa.* Westport, CT: Greenwood Press, 2004.

Suad, Joseph, ed. *Encyclopedia of Women and Islamic Cultures.* Vol. 3. Leiden: Brill, 2006.

Iran

Population: 79,853,900 (July 2013 est.)
Population Rank: 18th
Population Growth Rate: 1.24% (2013 est.)
Life Expectancy at Birth: 70.62 years (2013 est.)
Health Expenditures: 6% of GDP (2011)
People with Access to Safe Drinking Water: 96% of population (2010 est.)
Average Daily Caloric Consumption: 3,040
Adult Obesity Rate: 19.4% (2008)
Underweight Children under Age 5: 4.6% (2004)

The Iranian diet is particularly well balanced given that meat is eaten in relatively small proportion to vegetables and fruits, even when combined in the same dish. Sweets are eaten moderately, except during celebrations, and a variety of grains, in addition to rice and bread, including barley and whole-wheat germ, are consumed as well, providing additional sources of fiber.

According to the United Nations Food and Agriculture Organization, Iran's average proportions of dietary energy from protein (11%), fat (22%), and carbohydrates (67%) are desirable from a nutritional point of view. Food is considered a major part of health and well-being in Iran, not simply based on diet but based on its believed effect on personality and psychological well-being. A system of "hot" and "cold," called *garm* and *sard,* is similar to Ayurvedic and yin-yang principles of eating.

With a clear basis in seasonal availability the premise of garm and sard is an ancient one, believed to have originated thousands of years ago with Zoroaster, the founder of the Persian monotheistic religion of Zoroastrianism. The basis of the religion is the epic battle between good and evil, a battle that is thought to be waged within the human body and spirit as well. Foods must be used to balance the humors for best health, so, for example, if someone is "hot-natured," he or she must eat cold foods, and vice versa.

Garmi, or hotlike food, thickens weak blood and speeds up the metabolism, while *sardi,* or coldlike food, thins the blood and slows down the metabolism. It is important to note that those classifications have nothing to do with temperature or spiciness but rather a system that was developed millennia ago. Beef, for example, is "cold," while lamb is "hot." Duck is "hot," but turkey is "cold." Corn is "hot," but pumpkins are "cold," and so on. The classification applies to all manner of food, from meat to fish, fowl, grains, beans, vegetables, dairy, spices, herbs, and even beverages.

Ramin Ganeshram

Koreshte Geymeh

1/2 tsp saffron, dissolved in 1/3 c boiling water
1 tbsp olive oil or clarified butter
1 medium onion, thinly sliced,
2 lb lamb, cut into 1-in. cubes
1 tsp turmeric
1/2 tsp cinnamon
1 tsp salt
Freshly ground black pepper to taste
1 tbsp tomato paste
2 limou omani (dried Persian limes) or 1/4 c lemon juice
1/4 c split peas
4 small Yukon Gold potatoes, peeled and sliced into matchsticks
Canola oil, as needed, for frying potatoes

Dissolve the saffron in the boiling water and set aside for at least half an hour but preferably overnight. The longer it steeps, the darker the hue.

Heat the olive oil or butter in a Dutch oven or heavy-bottomed saucepan on medium-high heat and add the onion. Sauté the onion until translucent, about 3–4 minutes.

Add the lamb pieces to the onion mixture, and stir well. Fry until the lamb is browned on all sides, about 8–10 minutes.

Reduce the heat to medium low, and add the turmeric, cinnamon, salt, and pepper and cook, stirring, for 30 seconds. Add the tomato paste and mix well. Cook, stirring, for 3–4 minutes.

Add enough water to cover the lamb pieces by 2 inches and reduce heat to a simmer. Add the limou omani, if using, and simmer uncovered for 40 minutes. If using fresh lemon juice, add in the last 10 minutes of cooking.

While the lamb mixture is simmering, place the split peas in a small saucepan with enough water to cover. Simmer on medium-low heat for 20 minutes or until tender. Drain and set aside.

Heat a large frying pan with 2 inches of canola oil. Test the oil by adding one small potato stick. If it bubbles and fries, it is ready. Add the remaining potato sticks and fry until golden brown on all sides. Remove from the pan with a slotted spoon and place on a tray lined with paper towels or on a rack set over a sheet tray to drain.

Mix the split peas into the lamb mixture in the last 10 minutes of cooking.

Serve koreshte in a deep bowl or serving dish and arrange fried potato sticks on top of the stew.

Further Reading

Batmanglij, Najmieh. *New Food of Life: Ancient Iranian and Modern Persian Cooking and Ceremonies.* Waldorf, MD: Mage, 1992.

Shaida, Margaret. *The Legendary Cuisine of Persia.* New York: Interlink, 2002.

Iraq

Population: 31,858,481 (July 2013 est.)
Population Rank: 39th
Population Growth Rate: 2.29% (2013 est.)
Life Expectancy at Birth: 71.14 years (2013 est.)
Health Expenditures: 8.3% of GDP (2011)
People with Access to Safe Drinking Water: 79% of population (2010 est.)
Average Daily Caloric Consumption: Unknown
Adult Obesity Rate: 27% (2008)
Underweight Children under Age 5: 7.1% (2006)

It is difficult to generalize about the diet and health of the Iraqi people today as the country has been going through trying times for at least 20 years. Years of economic embargo and military attacks have left most of the population, especially children, malnourished. These adverse circumstances are also believed to be the cause for an increase in diseases, especially cancer, and environmental pollution.

Under normal circumstances, however, the Iraqi diet is reasonably healthy and balanced, with more emphasis on vegetables than meat, which is indeed mostly dictated by economic constraints rather than health concerns. The majority of cooks have embraced vegetable oil and abandoned saturated animal fats, such as *dihin hurr* (clarified butter) and liyya (sheep's tail fat). Still, most of the traditional foods, collectively called nawashif, are fried, a vice Iraqis share with other Middle Eastern cooks.

Dessert is not served after a meal on a daily basis. People are more accustomed to having dates and melon, for instance, than rich pastries. The favorite beverage to drink after meals is black tea, which indeed has been acknowledged to possess healthy properties. But people usually prefer to have it very sweet. While this might offset the tea's benefits, it does, nonetheless, satisfy the sweet tooth of many.

During medieval times, the predominant dietary theory in the region was influenced by the classical doctrine of the four elements, that is, that the world, including food and the human body, is basically composed of fire, air, water, and earth, each of which possesses innate qualities. For instance, fire is hot and dry, while water is cold and moist. To maintain good health, the elements need to be kept in harmonious balance. Although this theory is now obsolete, remnants of its practices can still be recognized in the way Iraqis look at food. For instance, gourds are considered an ideal summer vegetable because they are cold. People with short tempers should not consume eggplant in excess because it is hot. Iraqis eat a lot of dates, and to balance their hot properties, they are usually served with cucumber or yogurt, both of which are cold.

Nawal Nasrallah

Further Reading

Goldman, Rivka. *Mama Nazima's Jewish Iraqi Cuisine*. New York: Hippocrene Books, 2006.

Karim, Kay. *Iraqi Family Cookbook: From Mosul to America*. Falls Church, VA: Spi, 2006.

Nasrallah, Nawal. *Annals of the Caliphs' Kitchens: Ibn Sayyar al-Warraq's Tenth-Century Baghdadi Cookbook*. Leiden: Brill, 2007.

Nasrallah, Nawal. *Delights from the Garden of Eden: A Cookbook and a History of the Iraqi Cuisine*. 2nd ed. London: Equinox Books, 2010.

Israel

Population: 7,707,042 (July 2013 est.)
Population Rank: 97th
Population Growth Rate: 1.5% (2013 est.)
Life Expectancy at Birth: 81.17 years (2013 est.)

Health Expenditures: 7.7% of GDP (2011)
People with Access to Safe Drinking Water: 100% of population (2010 est.)
Average Daily Caloric Consumption: 3,540
Adult Obesity Rate: 26.2% (2008)
Underweight Children under Age 5: Unknown or Negligible

Overall, Israelis enjoy good health, and over 50 percent defined their health state as "very good" in a national survey. The life expectancy for women and men is 82 and 78.5 years, respectively. This is among the highest in the world. These statistics are commonly attributed to the national health care program, in which every citizen is insured and has access to primary care doctors, inexpensive medications, and hospitals. However, many health care

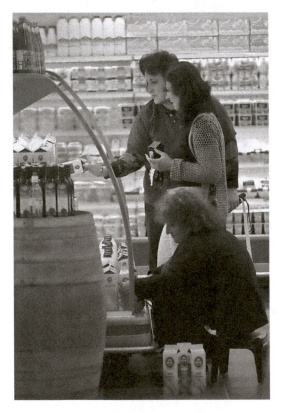

This large organic supermarket sells healthy food products in central Israel. (David Silverman/Getty Images)

professionals feel that Israelis, on the whole, do not practice healthy lifestyles and that the next generation of Israelis will suffer from considerably more chronic diseases than their parents. The once-healthy Israeli diet is rapidly deteriorating and is mimicking other developed countries that consume high quantities of processed foods, simple sugars, and saturated fats. Women in the workforce have less time to prepare home-cooked meals, and the availability of prepared products and fast food plays a large part in these dietary changes. Obesity is on the rise, and a disproportionate number of older Arab women are overweight. Along with dietary changes, Israelis are less active than ever before. Most families have cars, and the use of computers and television viewing are common nationwide. Fewer and fewer individuals work in jobs that require manual labor, and despite two to three years of army service for most young adults, the lifestyle is quite sedentary. There is a trend to increase physical activity for all ages, and health clubs are popular. However, only a small percentage (~20%) of the population actually exercises regularly.

Overnutrition does not guarantee adequate nutrients. Iron-deficiency anemia is not uncommon in small children, teens, and female adults. Surprisingly, in sunny Israel, vitamin D deficiency has also been documented. This is most evident in sectors of the population that dress modestly, including religious populations, both Muslim and Jewish, and Ethiopian women with dark skin and modest dress. Despite the availability of a wide variety of dairy products, calcium intake in every sector of the population has been shown to be significantly lower than recommended daily intakes.

There is great interest in the connection between diet and health, and most newspapers and magazines have columns reporting the most recent findings in nutritional research. Alternative eating practices such as vegetarianism, vegan diets, and fruitarianism are popular. Diet books written by local authors, but also translations of fads from around the world (Atkins, Blood Type, South Beach, and Weight Watchers) can be found in bookstores or purchased on the Internet. In addition, yoga lessons, Pilates, and Feldenkrais lessons are offered in studios and community centers. However, there is a large gap between the population's knowledge and their practices. There are definite attempts to improve nutritional consumption at both individual and national levels. Organic foods are available, and a wide selection of new products has been marketed by the food industry: eggs with omega-3 fatty acids; low-fat cheeses and mayonnaise; reduced-calorie cookies, crackers, and cereals; soy hotdogs, hamburgers, and tofu; whole-grain breads; and dietetic ice cream. This reflects the population's awareness of the connection between diet and health, but purchase of these products is not sufficiently widespread.

If supermarket shelf space reflects the consumption patterns of a community, soft drinks, candies, cookies, cakes, and salty snacks still fill a large proportion of market shelves. There are attempts by the Ministry of Health and the Ministry of Education to improve knowledge and attitudes regarding a healthy diet, but major changes still need to be made to improve the overall diet quality of the Israeli population.

Aliza Stark and Liora Gvion

Further Reading

Gurr, Janna. *The Book of New Israeli Food: A Culinary Journey.* Tel Aviv, Israel: Al Hashulchan Gastronomic Media, 2007.

Gvion, Liora. *Culinary Bridges versus Culinary Barriers: Social and Political Aspects of Palestinian Cookery in Israel.* Jerusalem: Carmel, 2006.

Kleinberg, Aviad, ed. *A Full Belly: Rethinking Food and Society in Israel.* [In Hebrew.] Tel Aviv, Israel: Keter, 2005.

Jordan

Population: 6,482,081 (July 2013 est.)
Population Rank: 104th
Population Growth Rate: 0.14% (2013 est.)
Life Expectancy at Birth: 80.3 years (2013 est.)
Health Expenditures: 8.4% of GDP (2011)
People with Access to Safe Drinking Water: 97% of population (2010 est.)
Average Daily Caloric Consumption: 2,980
Adult Obesity Rate: 30% (2008)
Underweight Children under Age 5: 1.9% (2009)

Before Jordan was a country, many people in the region were poorly nourished, unless they had herds or farms, but this was due to poverty and the scarcity of food, rather than flaws in the food traditions. As the country grew and food was more widely distributed, whether through aid, as at the beginning, or later, as the economy improved, the traditional diet was essentially wholesome, with a good balance of meat, dairy, vegetables, legumes, nuts, and fruit. Also, like other Mediterranean countries, Jordan relies heavily on olive oil in its cuisine. With increased urbanization, sugar consumption increased, which had its biggest impact on dental health. A bigger concern for most health organizations was the long-standing cultural encouragement of smoking.

Even today, approximately 62 percent of males smoke, though fewer than 10 percent of females smoke.

As with many countries, nutrition has declined with increased education, urbanization, and modernization, especially among the young. While fast food and soft drinks are not often consumed by adults or those in rural areas, they have been adopted by students in cities. In the past, the consumption of sweets was at least partially offset by a high consumption of dairy products, but with soft drinks increasingly replacing milk, health is suffering. Students who focus on fast food, modern snacks, and soft drinks are rarely getting enough vegetables and meat. Health organizations are making an effort to get nutrition programs into schools to help stop the deterioration of health.

Cynthia Clampitt

Fatush (Flatbread Salad)

Serves 6

1 pita
1 heart of romaine lettuce, shredded
2–3 tomatoes, roughly chopped
1 cucumber, peeled and cut into 1/4-in. chunks
3–4 scallions, white and light green parts, thinly sliced
1 sweet pepper, red or green, chopped
1/4 c chopped parsley
1/4 c chopped mint leaves
1 clove garlic
1 tsp salt
1 tbsp sumac
1/2 c lemon juice
1/2 c extra virgin olive oil
Freshly ground black pepper

Preheat oven to 400°F.

Cut the pita into approximately ¾-inch squares. Place on a baking sheet and toast in the oven until golden brown, about 8–10 minutes.

Put the lettuce, tomatoes, cucumber, scallions, sweet pepper, parsley, and mint in a bowl, and toss to combine.

Crush the garlic clove in a bowl with the salt and mix into a paste. Add the sumac and lemon juice, then whisk in the olive oil. Just before serving, add the toasted bread to the vegetables, pour the dressing over everything, and toss to combine. Chopped radishes or purslane are also common additions to this salad. Grind black pepper over to taste.

Further Reading

Abu-Jaber, Diana. *The Language of Baklava: A Memoir.* New York: Pantheon Books, 2005.

Bsisu, May S. *The Arab Table: Recipes and Culinary Traditions.* New York: William Morrow, 2005.

Robins, Philip. *A History of Jordan.* Cambridge: Cambridge University Press, 2004

Lebanon

Population: 4,131,583 (July 2013 est.)
Population Rank: 126th
Population Growth Rate: –0.04% (2013 est.)
Life Expectancy at Birth: 75.46 years (2013 est.)
Health Expenditures: 6.3% of GDP (2011)
People with Access to Safe Drinking Water: 100% of population (2010 est.)
Average Daily Caloric Consumption: 3,110
Adult Obesity Rate: 27.4% (2008)
Underweight Children under Age 5: 4.2% (2004)

The Lebanese diet is rich in fresh fruits and vegetables, so vitamin deficiency is not a serious problem. In particular, it uses lemon juice more abundantly than most cuisines. It also provides other healthful ingredients such as fish, nuts (which figure in the fillings of both pastries and stuffed vegetables), yogurt, and garlic.

Because of the availability of fish and olive oil, the Lebanese diet is lower in saturated fats and higher in omega-3 oils than that of some of its neighbors. However, although the Lebanese diet is the classic Mediterranean diet in many ways, sedentary city people tend to consume large amounts of sugar, butter, and refined wheat. Men who socialize in coffeehouses are at particular risk, because nothing but pastries is regularly served there, posing the danger of diabetes and cardiovascular problems. Many Lebanese are aware of these problems and explore health-food options.

Traditional medicinal concepts were derived from ancient Greek and Persian medicine and analyzed most complaints as due to an imbalance of the bodily humors. Medical treatments aimed to correct this supposed imbalance. All foods were held to have medicinal qualities, so medieval doctors often prescribed particular dishes—they even gave recipes, which cookbook writers eagerly plagiarized. These theories no longer exert much influence on diet, if any. Lebanon was the first Arab country to have modern medical schools, and it uses up-to-date pharmaceuticals and techniques. Folk remedies survive, however. Tea and yogurt are often recommended to those suffering from diarrhea, and mothers brew bitter medicinal teas for sick children.

Charles Perry

Further Reading

Heine, Peter. *Food Culture in the Near East, Middle East, and North Africa.* Westport, CT: Greenwood Press, 2004.

Malouf, Greg, Lucy Malouf, Anthony Bourdain, and Matt Harvey. *Saha: Chefs Journey through Lebanon.* Berkeley, CA: Periplus, 2007.

Palestinian Territories

Gaza Strip

Population: 1,763,387 (July 2013 est.)
Population Rank: 151st
Population Growth Rate: 3.01% (2013 est.)
Life Expectancy at Birth: 74.4 years (2013 est.)
Health Expenditures: Unknown
People with Access to Safe Drinking Water: Unknown
Average Daily Caloric Consumption: 2,130
Adult Obesity Rate: Unknown
Underweight Children under Age 5: Unknown or Negligible

West Bank

Population: 2,676,740 (July 2013 est.)
Population Rank: 141st
Population Growth Rate: 2.03% (2013 est.)
Life Expectancy at Birth: 75.46 years (2013 est.)
Health Expenditures: Unknown
People with Access to Safe Drinking Water: Unknown

Average Daily Caloric Consumption: 2,130
Adult Obesity Rate: Unknown
Underweight Children under Age 5: 2.2% (2007)

Various herbs and spices in Palestinian food are associated with health and well-being. Maramiyyeh (sage), *babunej* (chamomile), and za'atar (thyme) are all herbs that have medical applications to alleviate discomfort associated with stomach pains, colds, and so on. A number of medical practices are centered around the use of fenugreek, *hilbeh*. Hilbeh paste functions as a poultice for boils. An infusion of hilbeh leaves is sipped to ease digestive complaints such as inflammations and cramps. Stomach complaints are also addressed through the misnomer "white coffee," or *qahwa beyda,* an infusion of sweetened orange blossom water or rose water in hot water. This lacks any coffee—hence the whiteness alluded to in its name. Plants such as hilbeh have found their way into pharmaceutically produced capsules that are retailed to address glucose imbalance in older diabetic patients. Hilbeh seeds, when infused, are thought to ease menstrual pain and increase lactation in breast-feeding mothers. Cumin is noted as preventing flatulence, while za'atar, in its incarnations as both thyme and the dried mixture, is used in an infusion as a sore throat medicine, while combined with olive oil and rubbed on joints it is used to alleviate rheumatism. This same combination kept in a house augurs good fortune. An interesting sub-mythology adheres to za'atar: the dried powdered leaves, when consumed, will guarantee safety from serpents for 40 days.

Fiona Ross

Further Reading

Baramki, G. "Winter Traditions in Palestine." *This Week in Palestine,* Edition No. 106, February 2007.

Oleibo, A. "Tamarind, Tomatoes and Dried Yoghurt: The Aesthetics of the Palestinian Cuisine." *This Week in Palestine* 98 (June 2006).

Syria

Population: 22,457,336 (July 2013 est.)
Population Rank: 53rd
Population Growth Rate: 0.15% (2013 est.)
Life Expectancy at Birth: 75.14 years (2013 est.)
Health Expenditures: 3.7% of GDP (2011)

People with Access to Safe Drinking Water: 90% of population (2010 est.)
Average Daily Caloric Consumption: 3,050
Adult Obesity Rate: 27.1% (2008)
Underweight Children under Age 5: 10.1% (2009)

The Syrian diet is rich in fresh vegetables and notably in nuts, which figure in the fillings of both pastries and stuffed vegetables, so vitamin deficiency is not a serious problem. It is also rich in other healthful ingredients such as yogurt and garlic. However, it is low in fish and relatively high in saturated fats such as butter and lamb fat. This poses the danger of cardiovascular problems for sedentary city dwellers. At all levels of society, grain foods are a very important part of diet. Many urban men consume more simple than complex carbohydrates, because of the social institution of the coffeehouse and its tempting variety of baklavas.

Traditional medicinal concepts were derived from ancient Greek and Persian medicine; most complaints were analyzed as due to an imbalance of the bodily humors. Medical treatments aimed to correct this supposed imbalance. All foods were held to have medicinal qualities, so medieval doctors often prescribed particular dishes—they even gave recipes, which cookbook writers eagerly plagiarized. These theories no longer exert much influence on diet, and Syrian doctors now use modern medicines and techniques. Folk remedies survive, however. Tea and yogurt are often recommended to those suffering from diarrhea, and mothers brew bitter medicinal teas for sick children.

Charles Perry

Further Reading

Heine, Peter. *Food Culture in the Near East, Middle East, and North Africa.* Westport, CT: Greenwood Press, 2004.

Malouf, Greg, Lucy Malouf, Anthony Bourdain, and Matt Harvey. *Saha: Chefs Journey through Lebanon.* Berkeley, CA: Periplus, 2007.

Shoup, John A. *Culture and Customs of Syria.* Westport, CT: Greenwood Press, 2008.

Turkey

Population: 80,694,485 (July 2013 est.)
Population Rank: 17th
Population Growth Rate: 1.16% (2013 est.)
Life Expectancy at Birth: 73.03 years (2013 est.)

Health Expenditures: 6.7% of GDP (2011)
People with Access to Safe Drinking Water: 100% of population
Average Daily Caloric Consumption: 3,480
Adult Obesity Rate: 27.8% (2008)
Underweight Children under Age 5: 3.5% (2004)

The relation between food and health was central to Ottoman medicine both as a preventive measure and as a method of treatment. Ottoman medicine was based on Islamic medicine, which also followed the theories of the Greeks Hippocrates and Galen. Based on Galenic theory, as well as further knowledge developed by the Islamic physician İbn'i Sina (Avicenna) and the Andalusian botanist and pharmacist İbn-i Baytar, Ottoman medicine simply posited a direct causal connection between food and health. According to the system of thought, the human body has four humors or a combination of them, namely, blood, phlegm, yellow bile, and black bile, relating to the four elements of air, water, fire, and earth. Each represented qualities like hot, cold, moist, and dry. All foodstuffs carry these qualities, and one has to take care as to which combination of foods is to be consumed for one's health. This approach also gives much importance to seasonality, specifying what kinds of food have to be consumed to restore one's health.

This thought system is nowadays not known, but its influences still prevail. Turkish cuisine attaches much importance to seasonality and a balanced meal. Many dishes are automatically associated with seasons. A typical meal has a balanced distribution of proteins and carbohydrates and is accompanied by vegetables or wild greens. Two major healthy food items in Turkish cuisine are bulgur and yogurt. Bulgur is parboiled, dried, and cracked wheat berries, and this process enables the nutrients in the grain to be more easily absorbed. Dried fruit and nut snacks contribute to a healthy diet, along with the popular combination of *tahin-pekmez,* sesame paste and grape molasses.

Aylin Öney Tan

Further Reading

Bilgin, Arif, and Samancı Özge, eds. *Turkish Cuisine.* Ankara, Turkey: Ministry of Culture and Tourism Publications, 2008.

Halıcı, Nevin. *Nevin Halıcı's Turkish Cookbook.* London: Dorling Kindersley, 1989.

Halıcı, Nevin. *Sufi Cuisine.* London: Saqi Books, 2005.

Heine, Peter. *Food Culture in the Near East, Middle East, and North Africa.* Westport, CT: Greenwood Press, 2004.

Yemen and Oman

Yemen

Population: 25,408,288 (July 2013 est.)
Population Rank: 47th
Population Growth Rate: 2.5% (2013 est.)
Life Expectancy at Birth: 64.47 years (2013 est.)
Health Expenditures: 5.5% of GDP (2011)
People with Access to Safe Drinking Water: 55% of population (2010 est.)
Average Daily Caloric Consumption: 2,030
Adult Obesity Rate: 14.5% (2008)
Underweight Children under Age 5: 43.1% (2003)

Oman

Population: 3,154,134 (July 2013 est.)
Population Rank: 136th
Population Growth Rate: 2.06% (2013 est.)
Life Expectancy at Birth: 74.72 years (2013 est.)
Health Expenditures: 2.3% of GDP (2011)
People with Access to Safe Drinking Water: 89% of population (2010 est.)
Average Daily Caloric Consumption: Unknown
Adult Obesity Rate: 20.9% (2008)
Underweight Children under Age 5: 8.6% (2009)

Modern medicine has come to Oman and Yemen relatively recently. Traditional medicine included herbs, spices, and honey. Yemeni honey has a reputation for curing all ills, from sore throats to ulcers to insomnia. Both countries now have modern hospitals. Obesity is less of a problem in these two countries than in the rest of the peninsula, partly because Western influences have not been around so long and partly because of the use of qat, an appetite suppressant, in Yemen.

Christine Crawford-Oppenheimer

Zhug

This spicy mixture is popular in Yemen as a dip or a flavoring for stews. Yemenis believe it aids health and long life.

3 cardamom pods
1 tsp black peppercorns
1 tsp caraway seeds
4 hot chilies
1 c parsley
1 c fresh cilantro
6 cloves garlic
1 tsp ground cumin
$1/2$ tsp salt
$1/2$ tsp pepper
2 tbsp olive oil

With a blender or food processor, grind the first three ingredients. Add the remaining ingredients and blend into a coarse puree. Store the zhug in the refrigerator.

Further Reading

Dorr, Marcia S. *A Taste of Oman: Traditional Omani Food—Authentic Recipes and How to Prepare Them.* Muttrah, Oman: Mazoon, 1992.

Heine, Peter. *Food Culture in the Near East, Middle East, and North Africa.* Westport, CT: Greenwood Press, 2004.

Americas

Argentina

Population: 42,610,981 (July 2013 est.)
Population Rank: 32nd
Population Growth Rate: 0.98% (2013 est.)
Life Expectancy at Birth: 77.32 years (2013 est.)
Health Expenditures: 8.1% of GDP (2011)
People with Access to Safe Drinking Water: 97% of population (2008 est.)
Average Daily Caloric Consumption: 3,000
Adult Obesity Rate: 29.7% (2008)
Underweight Children under Age 5: 2.3% (2005)

Recently, Western health recommendations have become popular in Argentina, though it is difficult for these meat lovers to reduce their intake of meat and add more fish and vegetables to their diet. Those living in urban areas are more health conscious, and many avoid eating too much fat. The younger generations are great fans of American-style fast food, and visiting Starbucks, McDonald's, and Burger King has become a way of life for teenagers and young adults. Still, culinary traditions are very strong, and even though take-out sushi may be the rage at the moment, empanadas and choripán are still a part of the daily life of Argentineans.

Gabriela Villagran Backman

Chimichurri

1 c olive oil
1/3 c white wine vinegar
1/3 c finely chopped onion
3 finely chopped cloves garlic
1/2 tsp cayenne pepper
1 tsp dried oregano

> 1 tsp salt
> A pinch of black pepper
>
> Put the ingredients in a container with a lid, and blend well. Put in a cool place or in the refrigerator, and let the chimichurri rest for a couple of days so the flavors really blend. Serve as a sauce with barbecued meats and vegetables.

Further Reading

Foster, Dereck, and Richard Tripp. *Food and Drink in Argentina: A Guide for Tourists and Residents*. Buenos Aires: Aromas y Sabores, 2006.

Lovera, José Rafael. *Food Culture in South America*. Westport, CT: Greenwood Press, 2005.

Aruba and Bonaire

Population: 109,153 (July 2013 est.)
Population Rank: 190th
Population Growth Rate: 1.39% (2013 est.)
Life Expectancy at Birth: 76.14 years (2013 est.)
Health Expenditures: Unknown
People with Access to Safe Drinking Water: 100% of population (2010 est.)
Average Daily Caloric Consumption: 2,970
Adult Obesity Rate: Unknown
Underweight Children under Age 5: Unknown or Negligible

The chief diet and health concerns on Aruba center on obesity and diabetes. For the last 20 years insight and proactive plans have been sought. Focusing on youth, a program called Extreme H Games began. Long-term goals aim to teach children the impact of nutrition and physical activity on health. In 2008 the National Plan for Aruba (2009–18) for the Government of Aruba for the Fight against Overweight, Obesity, and Other Related Health Issues was launched. The plan was endorsed by the European Public Health Alliance in Brussels, Belgium.

Approximately 6 percent of all deaths are related to diabetes—with poor eating habits being targeted as the main cause. The improvement of these is suggested as the care and cure for 96 percent of cases. Increased consumption of simple and refined sugars and fried foods paired with a tendency toward little physical activity, or at least not enough to ward off this imbalance, contributes to this problem. With Aruba's inherent Arawak culture and love of dance—calypso, soca, merengue, and a mélange known as *socarengue*, vigorous dancing some might consider risqué, it seems possible that a revitalization of dance for all might hold the key to resolving both diet and health concerns.

Dorette Snover

Further Reading

Brushaber, Susan, and Arnold Greenburg. *Aruba, Bonaire, and Curacao: Alive.* Edison, NJ: Hunter, 2008.

Geddes, Bruce. *Lonely Planet. World Food Caribbean.* Oakland, CA: Lonely Planet, 2001.

Houston, Lynn Marie. *Food Culture in the Caribbean.* Westport, CT: Greenwood Press, 2005.

Barbados

Population: 288,725 (July 2013 est.)
Population Rank: 180th
Population Growth Rate: 0.34% (2013 est.)
Life Expectancy at Birth: 74.75 years (2013 est.)
Health Expenditures: 7.7% of GDP (2011)
People with Access to Safe Drinking Water: 100% of population (2010 est.)
Average Daily Caloric Consumption: 3,050
Adult Obesity Rate: 34.7% (2008)
Underweight Children under Age 5: Unknown or Negligible

Barbadians have always been known for their centenarians coming from all walks of life and from all financial sectors of the society. The problem now stands as to whether this reaching of such a ripe old age will continue, for it was attributed to the healthy diet before the influx of imported goods and fast-food outlets. Although Barbadians do lead a fairly healthy lifestyle compared to people who live in big cities, they are subjected to American cable television with its adoration of processed, unnatural, and fast foods. There is also the problem of pollution of the soil through the fertilizers and pesticides imported from the United States (in some cases those banned in that country); through the sudden massive amounts of construction of hotels and homes; and generally through the people's use of everything plastic, including foam containers for fast food, and bad waste and garbage practices.

Today, there is much concern about the diet and, therefore, the health of the average Barbadian. Heart disease, diabetes, and cancer are becoming almost the norm, and health and diet are in such question that government officials and those in the health care sector (doctors, nurses, etc.) have been finally forced into action. Far more information is available on keeping healthy, and an ever-growing number of people are following vegetarian or vegan diets, or simply eating less meat and more fish, fewer carbohydrates, and more greens and salads. However, the fight has only just begun.

Organic farmers are popping up, but the soil itself is still in question. Help has also come with the setting up of recycling plants and educational material on problems of pollution. Exercise is now becoming a priority for many, as can be seen on the various boardwalks on the south and west coast, around the Garrison (a race course in Christ Church), or simply in neighborhood streets or in the many gyms across the island. But there is still much work to be done.

Rosemary Parkinson

Further Reading

Elias, Marie Louise, and Josie Elias. *Barbados*. New York: Marshall Cavendish Benchmark, 2010.

Parkinson, Rosemary. *Culinaria: The Caribbean*. Cologne, Germany: Könemann, 1999.

Belize

Population: 334,297 (July 2013 est.)
Population Rank: 177th
Population Growth Rate: 1.97% (2013 est.)
Life Expectancy at Birth: 68.4 years (2013 est.)
Health Expenditures: 5.7% of GDP (2011)
People with Access to Safe Drinking Water: 98% of population (2010 est.)
Average Daily Caloric Consumption: 2,720
Adult Obesity Rate: 33.7% (2008)
Underweight Children under Age 5: 4.9% (2006)

Lifestyle diseases are common in Belize, especially heart disease, stroke, and diabetes. Today, many Belizeans, especially those of middle age, try to eat healthier although the most popular foods still contain too much sugar and saturated fat. The sudden death of the Belizean world music star Andy

Palacio from a heart attack in 2008 shocked the entire nation and dramatized the problem of a sedentary lifestyle and unhealthy diet. The influence of American relatives and mass media such as television on Belizean attitudes toward food and bodily health and appearance is also apparent, especially in more cosmopolitan places such as the capital Belmopan and Belize City, where even diet television dinners can be purchased at American-style supermarkets.

Lyra Spang and Richard Wilk

Further Reading

Jermyn, Leslie. *Belize*. New York: Marshall Cavendish, 2001.

Wilk, Richard R. *Home Cooking in the Global Village: Caribbean Food from Buccaneers to Ecotourists*. New York: Berg, 2006.

Bolivia

Population: 10,461,053 (July 2013 est.)
Population Rank: 82nd
Population Growth Rate: 1.63% (2013 est.)
Life Expectancy at Birth: 68.22 years (2013 est.)
Health Expenditures: 4.9% of GDP (2011)
People with Access to Safe Drinking Water: 88% of population (2010 est.)
Average Daily Caloric Consumption: 2,090
Adult Obesity Rate: 17.9% (2008)
Underweight Children under Age 5: 4.5% (2008)

Most Bolivians, particularly in the rural areas and low-income neighborhoods surrounding the large cities, lack access to basic medical care, with most sick people cared for by family members. While Bolivia has improving trends in terms of food supplies, these have not been sufficient to overcome widespread poverty, particularly in rural areas, and there is still a high incidence of hunger and malnutrition.

Many only partially understand and accept Western biomedical ideology and health care, as Bolivian health beliefs and practices typically revolve around rituals and ritual practitioners such as diagnostic specialists, curers, herbalists, and diviners. Divination, rituals, and ritual sacrifices are important in treating illness, as is the use of coca leaves, alcoholic beverages, and guinea pigs. Traditional medicine attaches importance to the social and supernatural etiology of illness and death, which often are attributed to strained social relations, witchcraft, or the influence of malevolent spirits. Dozens of illness categories, many psychosomatic, are recognized. Many curing rituals emphasize balanced, reciprocal relations with deities, who are "fed" and offered drink to dissipate illnesses.

The coca leaf is used extensively for traditional medicines for a supply of nutrients and natural energy. For high-altitude dwellers of the Andes, the leaf, when chewed or brewed into tea, acts as a palliative and stimulant, and a certain amount of cultivation is allowed for local use. Chewing of coca leaf is a common practice among peasant farmers, miners, laborers, and night workers. Soothsayers and indigenous priests use it in rituals passed down by their ancestors. And in many hotels in La Paz, foreign guests are welcomed with a cup of coca-leaf tea, which helps to relieve altitude sickness. Ancestral beliefs, confirmed by scientific research, credit coca-leaf chewing with alleviating hunger, fatigue, and sleepiness.

Bolivia has one of the highest infant mortality rates in South America and higher than anywhere else in Latin America—between 68 and 75 per 1,000 live births. Major causes of infant and child mortality include respiratory infections, diarrhea, and malnutrition; almost 30 percent of infants under age three suffer from chronic malnutrition. In Bolivia, more than one-quarter of infants are stunted. But between 1994 and 1998 the number of overweight women increased 9 percent, with the greatest increases seen among women with less education. Life expectancy is 68 years, compared to the Latin American average of 69. Indigenous women prefer to deliver at home because they do not feel confident in hospitals, mainly because their customs are ignored or denied in such health services.

In Bolivia, a culture of rural midwifery known as *partera* is adopted, where midwives speak the local language. Some of them understand the importance of evaluating risks, and for that purpose they use a sort of oracle, based in coca leaves. In traditional deliveries, women can choose the position. Most of them choose to squat, with their family around, and drink infusions of medicinal plants. Soon after the childbirth, women must keep warm and avoid contact with cold water.

Many projects supported by international organizations have been implemented over the past decades with very low success in terms of decreases in maternal mortality. Currently, the Bolivian government is developing a new strategy based on an intercultural reproductive health care approach, which incorporates the religious and traditional medicinal approach of the Bolivians with Western technologies and practices, uses the indigenous languages, takes advantage of the regional resources, and respects the habits and traditions of the people.

The annual expenditure for health care in Bolivia is $125 per capita. Health care providers are scarce, with only 3.2 physicians per 10,000 people and even fewer nurses. It has been estimated that 80 percent of the curable diseases in Bolivia are caused by polluted water. Although the country has abundant supplies of water, very little drinkable water is available to the people. Privatization of water delivery has resulted in price increases and "water wars" among providers.

Katrina Meynink

Further Reading

Hugo, R., A. Zubieta, B. McNelly, and C. Dunford. "Household Food Insecurity and Food Expenditure in Bolivia, Burkina Faso, and the Philippines." *Journal of Nutrition* 135, No. 5 (May 2006): 1431–37.

Larson, Brooke. "Unresolved Tensions: Bolivia Past and Present." *The Americas: A Quarterly Review of Inter-American Cultural History* 66, No. 1 (July 2009): 136–38.

Lovera, José Rafael. *Food Culture in South America.* Westport, CT: Greenwood Press, 2005.

Brazil

Population: 201,009,622 (July 2013 est.) (July 2013 est.)
Population Rank: 5th
Population Growth Rate: 0.83% (2013 est.)
Life Expectancy at Birth: 73.02 years (2013 est.)
Health Expenditures: 8.9% of GDP (2011)
People with Access to Safe Drinking Water: 98% of population
Average Daily Caloric Consumption: 3,450
Adult Obesity Rate: 18.8% (2008)
Underweight Children under Age 5: 2.2% (2007)

The Brazilian diet and consequently the population's health are guided by regional cultures and the different levels of economic development, which demonstrates a tremendous variation, although the country is 1 of the 10 most industrialized in the world. As Brazil's territory lies within several climate zones, there is not one single common diet, and there are also different food consumption levels, which depend on the highly heterogeneous availability of foods. People in the south plant extensive apple tree groves and will eat fruits and vegetables of European origin, such as spinach, red beets, lettuce, and carrots, to name a few. In the northeast, where the climate is drier, fruit consumption tends to be low, with the exception of the local tropical fruits, such as the wonderfully scented *seriguelas, pitombas, graviolas* (soursop fruit), and cashews.

It is important to notice that fruits play a very significant role in the local diets due to the variety of the species, whether native or introduced in the last 500 years. The same cannot be said of vegetables. Large areas do not consume them as part of their everyday lives. There is instead a preference for starches: potatoes, cassava, sweet potatoes, and yams as a side dish. A significant part of the northeast lies in a semiarid zone, where the climate resembles that of a desert. The Amazon rain forest is the northernmost region, and the Amazon territory also includes part of the Pantanal, the vast area of wetlands with seasonal inundations. Each region has its own specific plants and animals, both native and immigrant populations. Eating habits were influenced by the farm production of the colonial period and evolved according to the migration of people within Brazil, a constant event in Brazil's history. For instance, maté tea, which is a beverage in the pampas, the region that lies on the border with Uruguay and Argentina, is also widely consumed in Roraima, which lies on the border of Venezuela. This is due to the migration of people from the south to the far north as they followed the expansion of soybean plantations.

The preference for a specific type of bean might vary according to the region, but beans, which are full of iron, vitamin B, and amino acids, are a staple food all over Brazil, even though they are prepared in many different ways. Manioc flour is also produced and consumed from north to south, on the seacoast and in the countryside. Manioc flour is used in different ways, in both sweet and savory dishes, much like rice.

The fact that core nourishment is based on cooked beans, either accompanied by meat or, in very hard times, served with cassava flour, made it possible to avoid huge famines from historical times. Unfortunately, today their consumption is diminishing, and a new dietary parameter is establishing itself, more as a consequence of the country's urbanization and industrialization: high consumption of saturated fats and industrialized sugars, as well as a more sedentary life, resulting in a lower consumption of fresh vegetables and fruits, which are replaced by small industrialized snacks that are leading to obesity. The local dishes are losing importance in everyday life and more and more are turning into restaurant fare, as in most places in the Western world.

Marcia Zoladz

Grouper Moqueca

Serves 4

4 or 5 lb grouper or any fish that will not break up as it cooks
Juice of 1 lime
2 onions
1 red pepper
1 yellow pepper
1 jalapeño pepper
8 tomatoes, seeded
1 big garlic bulb
3 or 4 large basil leaves
8 sprigs fresh cilantro (optional)
1 bundle each parsley and chives
2 bay leaves
Salt to taste
Black pepper to taste

Ask the fishmonger to gut the fish and cut it crosswise into four or five large pieces, the head included.

At home, wash the grouper in running water, and rub it with the lime juice and a bit of salt. Place the pieces of fish side by side in a clay or iron pot big enough to fit all the pieces in one layer.

Shred and mix the peeled onions, the peppers (seeds and ribs removed), and the tomatoes in the food processor. Cover the fish with this mixture. Spread the herbs on the top, side, and bottom. Add the whole peeled garlic cloves. Place a lid on the pan and cook the stew at low temperature for roughly 15 minutes. The pieces of fish must remain covered with the sauce. Taste the sauce and add salt if necessary. Cook for 5 more minutes. Serve with white rice and pepper sauce.

Further Reading

Câmara Cascudo, Luís da. *História da Alimentação no Brasil*. 3rd ed. São Paulo, Brazil: Global Editora, 2004.

Zoladz, Marcia. "About Eggs, Two Countries and a Cake." In *Eggs in Cookery, Proceedings of the Oxford Symposium on Food and Cookery 2006*, edited by Richard Hosking, 322–32. Blackawton, UK: Prospect Books, 2007.

Zoladz, Marcia. "Cacao in Brazil or the History of a Crime." In *Food and Morality, Proceedings of the Oxford Symposium on Food and Cookery 2007*, edited by Susan Friedland, 309–20. Blackawton, UK: Prospect Books, 2008.

Canada

Population: 34,568,211 (July 2013 est.)
Population Rank: 37th
Population Growth Rate: 0.77% (2013 est.)
Life Expectancy at Birth: 81.57 years (2013 est.)
Health Expenditures: 11.2% of GDP (2011)
People with Access to Safe Drinking Water: 100% of population
Average Daily Caloric Consumption: 3,530
Adult Obesity Rate: 26.2% (2008)
Underweight Children under Age 5: Unknown or Negligible

Canadians have a culture of eating "pioneer" food—high protein, high fat, high carbohydrates—and lots of it. This pattern dates back to the relatively recent settling of the land, and the hardworking rural and farm population. Now, only a fraction—less than 1 percent—of the population lives on farms. But some Canadians eat as if they still routinely drive a horse-drawn plow (which they do not).

Health Canada, a branch of the Canadian government, is entrusted with Canadians' good food and nutrition. The Canadian government calls maintaining the safety of the country's food supply a "shared responsibility" among government, industry, and consumers, based on what it calls evidence-based nutrition policies and standards. These policies and standards are reflected in Canada's Food Guide. The guide makes recommendations by suggesting food options rather than daily allowances of nutrients. Offering choices from four basic food groups is intended to supply Canadians with the proper intake of nutrients, but it does not account for the specific needs of all individuals, such as women who need more iron.

Furthermore, Health Canada recommends to Canadian consumers that they eat at least one dark green and one orange vegetable each day; have vegetables and fruit more often than juice; make at least half of grain products whole grain each day; drink skim, 1 percent, or 2 percent milk each day; have meat alternatives such as beans, lentils, and tofu often; eat at least two Food Guide servings of fish each week; include a small amount of unsaturated fat each day; and, lastly, satisfy their thirst with water. These messages do not seem to be getting through to the public, though.

Despite—or perhaps because of—Canadians' limited adherence to health precepts, new crops aimed at better health are constantly being monitored, trialed, and introduced into the food system. Value-added crops continue to be an area of exciting development, particularly those with health benefits. For example, Canadian-grown oilseeds such as canola, sunflower, and flax are known today for their health benefits, and the industry has successfully developed a strong market based on these qualities. Canola was developed in Canada and is often the nation's most valuable crop, with annual exports of canola seed, oil, and meal valued at more than CDN$3 billion. Canola is an achievement of Canada's research community and is a testament to how responding to consumer demands for quality and nutrition pays big dividends over time. Canadian wheat is renowned the world over for its quality as well. Looking into the future, an organization called the Advanced Foods and Materials Network is Canada's front line of research and development in the area of advanced foods and biomaterials, including improved frozen-food quality and reduced salt intake.

Owen Roberts, Rebecca Moore, and Anita Stewart

Further Reading

Duncan, Dorothy. *Canadians at Table: Food, Fellowship, and Folklore. A Culinary History of Canada.* Toronto, ON: Dundurn, 2006.

Hamilton, Janice. *Canada.* Minneapolis, MN: Lerner, 2008.

Chile

Population: 17,216,945 (July 2013 est.)
Population Rank: 62nd
Population Growth Rate: 0.86% (2013 est.)
Life Expectancy at Birth: 78.27 years (2013 est.)
Health Expenditures: 7.5% of GDP (2011)
People with Access to Safe Drinking Water: 96% of population (2010 est.)
Average Daily Caloric Consumption: 2,960
Adult Obesity Rate: 29.4% (2008)
Underweight Children under Age 5: 0.5% (2008)

Chile's traditional diet—the blend of indigenous foods and those introduced by the Spanish—forms the basis of a diet with plenty of fruits and vegetables,

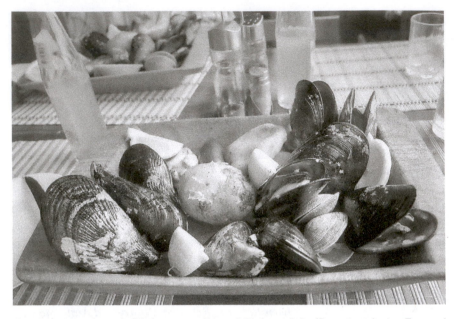

Curanto, based on shellfish, is a traditional Chilean dish. (Francisco Javier Espuny/
Dreamstime.com)

legumes, grains, dairy foods, abundant seafood, and some meat. Until the late
twentieth century, many Chileans practiced this variation of the nutrient-
dense, lower-fat Mediterranean diet coupled with a lifestyle that brought families together at the table for meals. During the midday meal break from 1 to
4 p.m., offices and schools closed, giving a relaxing break from school and
work. At the same time, among Chile's poorest citizens, malnutrition and
infant mortality were high.

Chile's growing economic prosperity from the 1990s on fueled a radical
change in eating habits across the entire population. Malnutrition practically
disappeared, infectious diseases decreased, and life expectancy increased to
one of the highest in South America. The Chilean story is similar to the one
in many countries where the abandonment of traditional foods and lifestyle
choices and the choice of more highly processed foods and faster-paced urban
lives have been followed by an increase in childhood obesity (at 20.8% for
primary-school students in 2008) and risk for cardiovascular disease. Heart
disease is the cause of 28 percent of deaths, topping all other causes.

Chronic illness, including high blood pressure and obesity related to cardiovascular disease, increased significantly. Researchers are limited by the

fact that Chile does not collect nationwide nutrition data. They rely on targeted studies, including a 2003 *National Health Survey* reporting that 38 percent of adult Chileans were overweight and 23 percent were obese, with higher rates among women and in lower socioeconomic groups. A third of Chileans had high blood pressure.

Chileans are selecting more energy-dense foods and meat for an average 25 percent increase in both calorie and fat consumption between 1988 and 1998. Per capita consumption of soft drinks and tea is among the highest in the world. More people in Chile have moved to the cities, and rates of alcohol and drug abuse have increased. Add to that the high incidence of smoking (42% of adults) and the serious air pollution in Santiago, one of Latin America's most polluted cities. Chileans are also not keen to exercise: 90 percent of adult Chileans report a sedentary lifestyle.

One unusual finding in Chile's nutrition transition has been among the indigenous rural populations, who continue a traditional diet along with plenty of physical activity growing crops and tending animals. Despite being among the poorest of Chileans, the Mapuche in southern Chile and the Aymara in the north have each been found to have a very low incidence of diabetes. However, when the Mapuche move to an urban setting (about 60% of Mapuche are urbanites), the numbers of diabetics doubles from 4.1 to 9.8 percent, as does obesity. Among the rural Aymara, the incidence of diabetes was 1 percent. Researchers are intrigued because, unlike the rural Aymara and Mapuche, North American Indians, rural as well as urban, have epidemic rates of diabetes. Preliminary data point to the preventive effect of the traditional diet and the activity it takes to produce it.

Chile does have a well-established national public health system with a succession of rural posts, public health centers, and hospitals. Since the mid-1990s, those involved in nutrition programs and academia have been actively advocating to better link that system with a stronger nutrition policy. Through that system, health-promotion messages have increased across the country, and programs have begun in schools to promote exercise and better eating habits. Advocates are pushing for laws to restrict advertising for cigarettes and alcohol and to limit advertising for energy-dense, nutrient-poor foods on television, especially during children's prime viewing times.

Mary Gunderson

Further Reading

Freire, Wilma. *Nutrition and an Active Life: From Knowledge to Action*. Washington, DC: Pan American Health Organization, Regional Office of the World Health Organization, 2005.

Lovera, José Rafael. *Food Culture in South America*. Westport, CT: Greenwood Press, 2005.

Colombia

Population: 45,745,783 (July 2013 est.)
Population Rank: 29th
Population Growth Rate: 1.1% (2013 est.)
Life Expectancy at Birth: 75.02 years (2013 est.)
Health Expenditures: 6.1% of GDP (2011)
People with Access to Safe Drinking Water: 92% of population
Average Daily Caloric Consumption: 2,660
Adult Obesity Rate: 17.3% (2008)
Underweight Children under Age 5: 3.4% (2010)

The most famous living Colombian artist, Fernando Botero, famously portrays his countrymen as pudgy sensualists who are obsessed with food. His sometimes cruel, sometimes sympathetic portraits are an exaggeration of a fact; a 1999 study showed that over 40 percent of the country's citizens are obese, and that figure may be rising. It is ironic that a government that has historically focused on getting its rural and native citizens enough to eat now must change its focus to convincing them to switch to healthier foods. The popularity of sugary sodas and a diet heavy in meat, coconut milk, and cream, plus the increasing use of motor vehicles instead of walking for everyday tasks, are probably to blame. Colombians who can afford it often get weight-loss surgery rather than change their diets, and more of these operations are performed there than anywhere else in South America.

When Colombians do fall ill, traditional practices that are based on a diet of scarcity are actually counterproductive. Traditional ideas of health prescribe aguapanela, the mix of sugarcane juice and water, for almost any illness, and especially in diabetic people this can make things much worse. Colombians also ascribe characteristics of hot and cold to many foods and give beef broth the kind of reverence accorded to chicken soup in eastern European cultures.

There is a specific regimen called the *dieta* that mothers are supposed to observe for 40 days after giving birth. Besides never being exposed to direct sun, a new mother is supposed to eat sancocho and hot chocolate; at the end of this period, she takes a bath in herbs before going outside and resuming normal life. If the baby becomes sick at any time, putting slices of cucumber on its head is supposed to help protect it from sinus infection.

The influence of Colombian traditional healers has been growing, and the commercialization of their remedies based on Amazonian plants has been a boon for people who want to preserve jungle regions. Colombian culture is very macho, and there are many recipes for aphrodisiacs. Some of these involve eating insects such as leafcutter ant queens, a logical choice for someone obsessed with fertility, since ant queens are literally egg machines. Since leafcutter ant queens are high in protein and have low levels of saturated fat, this at least does no harm, unlike more toxic alternatives.

Richard Foss

Sopa de Frijoles Canarios (Canary Bean Soup)

Serves 6–8

This is a traditional Colombian dish. Sazón preparado is a popular seasoning mix throughout the Caribbean. The Goya brand is most popular in Colombia, but it contains more monosodium glutamate than many other versions.

1 garlic clove
$1/4$ c onion, chopped
$1/4$ c red bell pepper, chopped
$1/4$ c green pepper, chopped
1 scallion, chopped
1 lb canary beans (or kidney, pinto, or cranberry beans), soaked overnight
2 lb pork ribs, cut into pieces
14 c water
2 c grated carrots
1 cube chicken bouillon
$1/2$ tbsp ground cumin
$1/2$ tbsp sazón preparado with saffron
$1/2$ c chopped cilantro
1 large potato, peeled and diced
Salt and pepper

In a food processor, combine garlic, onion, red bell pepper, green pepper, and scallion and process until finely chopped.

In a large pot over medium heat, combine the processed vegetables, beans, pork ribs, water, carrots, and chicken bouillon. Slightly cover and simmer for 1 1/2 hours.

Add the ground cumin, sazón preparado, cilantro, and potato. Simmer for 30–40 minutes more, or until the beans are tender.

Season with salt and pepper. Serve with white rice and hot sauce on the side.

Further Reading

Karpf, Helln. *The Cuisine of Cartagena de Indias: Legacy of Spanish Cooking in Colombia.* Santa Fe de Bogotá, Colombia: Ediciones Gamma, 2001.

Montaña, Antonio. *A Taste of Colombia.* Bogotá, Colombia: Villegas, 2001.

Costa Rica

Population: 4,695,942 (July 2013 est.)
Population Rank: 121st
Population Growth Rate: 1.27% (2013 est.)
Life Expectancy at Birth: 78.06 years (2013 est.)
Health Expenditures: 10.9% of GDP (2011)
People with Access to Safe Drinking Water: 97% of population (2010 est.)
Average Daily Caloric Consumption: 2,810
Adult Obesity Rate: 23.7% (2008)
Underweight Children under Age 5: 1.1% (2009)

The Costa Rican diet, grounded in a protein-laden rice-and-bean mix and supplemented by proteins from meats, eggs, and cheeses, as well as fruits and vegetables, seems quite healthy, aside from a tendency to prefer frying over other cooking methods. Additionally, Costa Ricans favor generous portions at lunch and breakfast, and light dinners. A simple diet combined with a national health care system fosters a relatively healthy population. Costa Rica even boasts one of the longest-living communities in the world, in the country's northern province, Guanacaste.

Nonetheless, changes in lifestyles and increases in unhealthy globalized foodways have spurred health concerns. Costa Ricans complain of constant gastritis and constipation. Better infrastructure and access to cars and public transportation mean that many Costa Ricans do not benefit from daily exercise. Recently, gyms and workout classes have come into fashion, but not all socioeconomic classes can afford such luxuries. Instead, rates of dieting, eating disorders, and self-medication with expensive medicines and health products are growing. A discourse of healthy eating and favoring natural foods and medicine has grown in the media and on the ground, though practices are slower to follow.

Theresa Preston-Werner

Further Reading

Preston-Werner, Theresa. "*Gallo Pinto:* Tradition, Memory, and Identity in Costa Rican Foodways." *Journal of American Folklore* 122, No. 483 (2009): 11–27.

Preston-Werner, Theresa. "In the Kitchen: Negotiating Changing Family Roles in Costa Rica." *Journal of Folklore Research* 45, No. 3 (2008): 329–59.

Ross González, Marjorie. *Entre el comal y la olla: Fundamentos de gastronomía costarricense.* San José, Costa Rica: Editorial Universidad Estatal a Distancia, 2006.

Cuba

Population: 11,061,886 (July 2013 est.)
Population Rank: 77th
Population Growth Rate: –0.13% (2013 est.)
Life Expectancy at Birth: 78.05 years (2013 est.)
Health Expenditures: 10% of GDP (2011)
People with Access to Safe Drinking Water: 94% of population (2010 est.)
Average Daily Caloric Consumption: 3,300
Adult Obesity Rate: 21.5% (2008)
Underweight Children under Age 5: 3.4% (2000)

Recently, in Cuba, the government has tried to encourage people to eat more vegetables and less fatty foods. Many Cubans claim that this is very hard for them, as they have grown accustomed to eating fried foods and a lot of pork, which can be a very fatty meat. For a long time fresh vegetables were hard to find in Cuba, so many Cubans are not used to eating vegetables daily. However, fresh fruits have always been an important part of a healthy Cuban diet, and most Cubans eat several servings of fruit every day. Nearly all of the grains Cubans eat—mostly rice—are refined grains. The white rice that is eaten daily has far less nutrients in it than brown rice would; however, brown rice is nearly impossible to find in Cuba and, even if it were, Cubans are not accustomed to eating it.

In addition to encouraging healthier eating, the Cuban government encourages Cubans to get plenty of exercise and take part in healthy physical activity. Eating more fresh vegetables and exercising daily is thought to help reduce the chances of getting heart disease or acquiring other related health problems.

Hanna Garth

Further Reading

Benjamin, Medea, Joseph Collins, and Michael Scott. *No Free Lunch: Food and Revolution in Cuba Today.* Princeton, NJ: Princeton University Press, 1984.

Funes, Fernando, Luis Garcia, Martin Bourque, and Nilda Perez. *Sustainable Agriculture and Resistance: Transforming Food Production in Cuba.* Oakland, CA: Food First Books, 2001.

Curaçao and Sint Maarten

Curaçao

Population: 146,836 (July 2013 est.)
Population Rank: 188th
Population Growth Rate: Unknown
Life Expectancy at Birth: 76.25 years (2009 est.)
Health Expenditures: Unknown
People with Access to Safe Drinking Water: Unknown
Average Daily Caloric Consumption: 2,970
Adult Obesity Rate: Unknown
Underweight Children under Age 5: Unknown or Negligible

Pork- and fat-laden "resort" food is consumed on Curaçao and Sint Maarten. It is recommended that locals return to their original foods and seafood and avoid the trap of fast foods, which, while quicker to consume, also pose greater health and long-term risks as well as leading to a loss of food culture. When eaten, chicken, goat, and iguana are high in protein and, depending on the cooking method, may contain less fat. As on many of the Dutch Antilles, iguanas are now protected and are now often raised on farms instead of depleting the already-challenged wild population.

Irish moss is a beverage consumed for health and aphrodisiac purposes. It is made with Malta, a nonalcoholic beverage, and a seaweed. It is thought to aid in the cure of bronchitis, tuberculosis, and intestinal dilemmas. Ginger beer is often offered as a tonic for digestion and menstrual cramps and as an alternative to aspirin.

Dorette Snover

Further Reading

Besson, Jean. "A Paradox in Caribbean Attitudes to Land." In *Land and Development in the Caribbean*, edited by Jean Besson and Janet Momsen, 13–45. London: Macmillan, 1987.

Brathwaite, Kamau. *Roots*. Ann Arbor: University of Michigan Press, 1993.

Brushaber, Susan, and Arnold Greenburg. *Aruba, Bonaire, and Curaçao: Alive*. Edison, NJ: Hunter, 2002.

Houston, Lynn Marie. *Food Culture in the Caribbean*. Westport, CT: Greenwood Press, 2005.

Dominica

Population: 73,286 (July 2013 est.)
Population Rank: 201st
Population Growth Rate: 0.22% (2013 est.)
Life Expectancy at Birth: 76.39 years (2013 est.)
Health Expenditures: 5.9% of GDP (2011)
People with Access to Safe Drinking Water: 95% of population (2010 est.)
Average Daily Caloric Consumption: 3,110
Adult Obesity Rate: 24.9% (2008)
Underweight Children under Age 5: Unknown or Negligible

The nutritious local food, the use of herbal remedies and bush teas, the more traditional methods of cooking, and Dominica's clean natural environment, which is more conducive to a healthy lifestyle, all contribute to the island's fast-growing reputation as a center for mental and physical well-being.

The high ratio of healthy centenarians per capita is testimony to this.

But there is doubt whether this phenomenon will last very much longer, as the lifestyle of younger Dominicans is changing and many do not lead the same active lifestyle as their parents and grandparents or follow the same healthy diet. Tobacco smoking is on the increase, as is drug and alcohol abuse. Food imports are also on the rise, as local food production has begun to decline. The largely unregulated diversion of former agricultural land into real estate development raises concerns about the nation's long-term ability to feed itself.

The prevalence of noncommunicable diseases is rising. Stroke, heart disease, diabetes, and cancer account for a high percentage of deaths. Initiatives such as healthy eating campaigns, screenings, and government proposals to combat noncommunicable diseases, as well as organizations like the recently established Dominica Organic Agriculture Movement, will likely help reduce some of the underlying causes of ill health.

Celia Sorhaindo and Rosemary Parkinson

Crab Backs

$1/4$ c oil
$1/2$ tbsp soy sauce
2 cloves fresh garlic, grated
1 large onion, finely chopped
2 mild chili peppers, finely chopped
1 stalk fresh celery, finely chopped
1 sprig parsley, finely chopped
5 sprigs chives, finely chopped
2 sprigs thyme, finely chopped
1 tbsp lime juice
$3/4$ lb crabmeat, fresh or canned
2 tbsp tomato paste
1 hot Scotch bonnet pepper, seeded and finely chopped
3 tbsp breadcrumbs
Salt and black pepper to taste
6 crab back shells, cleaned and scrubbed

Heat oil in a deep frying pan. Add soy sauce, garlic, onion, chili peppers, celery, parsley, chives, and thyme. Stir and let steam for just a few seconds. Add lime juice. Let steam for another 5 minutes. Add enough water to cover ingredients. Add all the crabmeat. Stir. Add tomato paste and hot pepper, and sprinkle breadcrumbs over the mixture, stirring constantly until a good thick consistency is reached. More crabmeat than bread-crumbs is preferred. Add salt and pepper to taste. Reduce heat. Let steam for another 2 minutes just to get rid of excess water. Place mixture into crab backs, sprinkle with more breadcrumbs, and brown under a grill just before serving. Crab backs can also be prepared and frozen; when ready for use, remove from freezer, defrost, and use same way as described. Serve with a sprig of parsley as garnish. Two crab backs are usually served per person.

Further Reading

Crask, Paul. *Dominica—Bradt Travel Guide*. Chalfont St. Peter, UK: Bradt Travel Guides, 2008.

Parkinson, Rosemary. *Culinaria: The Caribbean*. Cologne, Germany: Könemann, 1999.

Dominican Republic

Population: 10,219,630 (July 2013 est.)
Population Rank: 85th
Population Growth Rate: 1.28% (2013 est.)
Life Expectancy at Birth: 77.62 years (2013 est.)
Health Expenditures: 5.4% of GDP (2011)
People with Access to Safe Drinking Water: 86% of population (2010 est.)
Average Daily Caloric Consumption: 2,260
Adult Obesity Rate: 21.2% (2008)
Underweight Children under Age 5: 3.4% (2007)

Type 2 diabetes is prevalent in the population of the Dominican Republic. This is no doubt aggravated by diets high in rice, sugar, starchy roots, fatty meats, and sugars from many fresh fruits. Additionally, dietary problems in the Dominican Republic tended to be concentrated in the areas of deficiencies in iodine, vitamin A, and iron, and approximately 5 percent of school-age children have goiter problems. The severity varies regionally, and the World Health Organization has enforced use of iodized salt in cooking since 1920.

Marty Martindale

Further Reading

Drago, Lorena. *Beyond Rice and Beans: The Caribbean Latino Guide to Eating Healthy with Diabetes*. Alexandria, VA: American Diabetes Association, 2006.

Gonzalez, Clara, and Ilana Benady. *Traditional Dominican Cookery*. Santo Domingo, Dominican Republic: Lunch Club Press, 2005.

Ecuador

Population: 15,439,429 (July 2013 est.)
Population Rank: 67th
Population Growth Rate: 1.4% (2013 est.)
Life Expectancy at Birth: 76.15 years (2013 est.)
Health Expenditures: 7.3% of GDP (2011)
People with Access to Safe Drinking Water: 94% of population (2010 est.)
Average Daily Caloric Consumption: 2,300
Adult Obesity Rate: 21.4% (2008)
Underweight Children under Age 5: 6.2% (2004)

Ecuador is a country of great disparities in income and food security. While a privileged minority enjoys general good nutrition and health, a significant proportion of the indigenous rural population as well as the urban poor is undernourished. This has partly been the result of failed government policies to implement equitable food distribution, but it means that iron-deficiency anemia is a serious problem and as many as 15 percent of children's growth is stunted. There is also an extremely high infant mortality rate. Water-borne illnesses are a serious problem, and many people have no access to clean water. Parasites are also a problem, as are malaria, hepatitis, and typhoid.

Ken Albala

Further Reading

Archetti, Eduardo P., and Valentina Napolitano. *Guinea Pigs: Food, Symbol and Conflict of Knowledge in Ecuador.* New York: Berg, 2001.

Weismantel, Mary J. *Food, Gender and Poverty in the Ecuadorian Andes.* Philadelphia: University of Pennsylvania Press, 1988.

El Salvador

Population: 6,108,590 (July 2013 est.)
Population Rank: 107th
Population Growth Rate: 0.29% (2013 est.)
Life Expectancy at Birth: 73.93 years (2013 est.)
Health Expenditures: 6.8% of GDP (2011)
People with Access to Safe Drinking Water: 88% of population (2010 est.)
Average Daily Caloric Consumption: 2,590
Adult Obesity Rate: 25.8% (2008)
Underweight Children under Age 5: 6.6% (2008)

The general diet of El Salvador, which consists of corn and beans supplemented with meat, dairy, and fresh produce, is healthy. Tortillas and beans provide more than enough complex protein for the body; beans provide fiber, magnesium, and vitamin B, among other nutrients, and tortillas gain zinc and iron from being ground on a grinding stone. Tropical fruits that are native to El Salvador, such as mangoes, bananas, sour oranges, and papayas, offer plenty of carotenoids and vitamin C.

With almost half of the population living below the national poverty level, financial distress often prevents families from getting a well-balanced, healthy diet in El Salvador. Fresh fruits and meats like beef and chicken are not affordable to all income levels, and the little meat purchased by the poor tends to be high in fat and low in nutrition, like sausages. Food security in El Salvador has been threatened by natural disasters (including an earthquake and a mudslide), rising food prices, little education, lack of food production, and financial hardship. Sixteen percent of rural families do not make enough money to buy food. A civil war in the 1980s displaced rural communities that had been relied on to produce cereals for the country, which has led to reduced food supplies. Malnutrition in children under the age of five has led to an increase in stunted growth among Salvadoran children.

Leena Trivedi-Grenier

Cheese-Stuffed Pupusas

Serves 4 (1 pupusa each)

Dough
2 c masa harina
1 c water
1 tbsp olive oil
Salt and pepper to taste
Filling
1/2 c crumbled queso fresco (fresh cheese)
1/2 c white melting cheese, like Chihuahua

Mix the masa harina, water, and olive oil in a bowl until combined into a soft dough. Taste for flavor, and then adjust seasonings with salt and pepper to your preference.

Split the dough into 8 evenly sized balls, roughly 2 inches in diameter. Roll out each ball into a 6-inch circle. Sprinkle cheese evenly over the middle of the tortilla, then top with another rolled-out tortilla, pinching the edges to seal the filling inside. Place the stuffed tortilla on a preheated ungreased griddle, and cook on both sides until the tortilla is crispy and the cheese is melted and warm, a few minutes.

Further Reading

Balladares-Castellon, Enrique. "Central America." *Encyclopedia of Food and Culture*, edited by Solomon H. Katz, 1:340–46. New York: Gale Cengage, 2003.

McDonald, Michael R. *Food Culture in Central America*. Westport, CT: Greenwood Press, 2009.

French Guiana

See France entry for statistical information

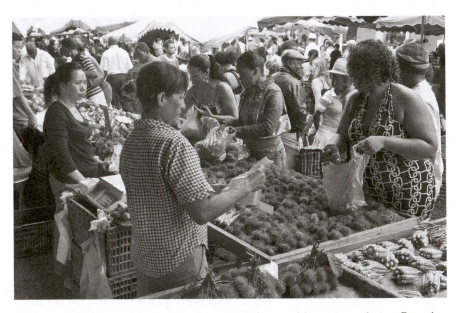

Members of the Hmong people sell fruits and vegetables at a market in French Guiana. The Hmong have largely achieved economic independence through market farming. (Jody Amiet/AFP/Getty Images)

The French Guianese diet is rich in fresh fruits and vegetables and seafood, yet with a poor economy, some may not have access to a healthy, balanced diet. Relying too heavily on inexpensive starches, such as rice, could deprive one of important nutrients and lead to malnutrition, especially among children. With the country's geography, access to a safe water supply is also an issue. The country's status as a French overseas department means that the population has access to health care that otherwise would not be available, including implementation of public health services and health education.

The Hmong, in the smaller villages, have been able to maintain some of their traditional ways of life and culture, including religious beliefs such as shamanism, even if they have converted to Christianity. Appeals to shamans for improving health often involve animal sacrifices. The Hmong are also fairly healthy, growing and eating their own fruits and vegetables and keeping fit through the physical demands of farming.

Erin Laverty

Further Reading

Crosby, Alfred W., Jr. *The Columbian Exchange: Biological and Cultural Consequences of 1492*. Westport, CT: Praeger, 2003.

Skelton, Tracey, ed. *Introduction to the Pan-Caribbean*. New York: Oxford University Press, 2004.

Grenada

Population: 109,590 (July 2013 est.)
Population Rank: 189th
Population Growth Rate: 0.52% (2013 est.)
Life Expectancy at Birth: 73.55 years (2013 est.)
Health Expenditures: 6.2% of GDP (2011)
People with Access to Safe Drinking Water: 94% of population (2000 est.)
Average Daily Caloric Consumption: 2,420
Adult Obesity Rate: 22.5% (2008)
Underweight Children under Age 5: Unknown or Negligible

Despite the arrival of fast-food franchises in Grenada, the typical diet is a healthy one. Fresh fruits, vegetables, and ground provisions have not yet become foods that are scorned by the young in favor of hamburgers and southern fried chicken. With fishing villages along the coastlines of all three islands, fresh seafood is also a healthy staple of the Grenadian diet. Combine this fresh food with sunshine and the great outdoors and there is no reason why anyone should put on too many extra pounds—though some of those wonderful restaurant desserts may indeed prove too much to resist.

Paul Crask and Rosemary Parkinson

Grenadian Oil-Down

3 dry coconuts or 6 cans coconut milk
1-in. × 2-in. piece fresh turmeric, peeled and grated
$1/2$ c vegetable oil
2 lb chicken wings
1 lb salt fish, soaked in water overnight
1 salted pig tail, whole
6 green bananas, peeled and cut in half
1 whole breadfruit, peeled and cut into chunks
12 medium-sized leaves of callaloo bush
1 leaf chadon bennie (also known as shadow-bennie), finely chopped (or a handful of cilantro can be used instead)
4 onions, peeled and finely chopped
6 cloves garlic, finely chopped
3 sprigs parsley, finely chopped
6 stalks fresh chives, finely chopped
3 leaves broad-leaf thyme, finely chopped
4 fresh mint leaves, finely chopped
6 leaves fresh basil, finely chopped
1 red hot pepper or Scotch bonnet, seeded and finely chopped
2 red hot peppers or Scotch bonnets, whole
2 seasoning peppers, finely chopped
1–2 tbsp butter
Salt and pepper to taste
Dumplings
2 c flour
$1/2$ c butter
1 tsp salt
1 tsp ground cinnamon

Break the coconuts, and remove and grate the hard interior white flesh. Add the turmeric to the grated flesh. Pour hot water over this mixture and squeeze through a muslin bag until all the coconut milk has been extracted. When substituting this method with 6 cans of coconut milk (unsweetened), add the turmeric, bring to a boil, and still put the liquid through a sieve in order to remove the grated turmeric, just keeping the coloring, which should be a bright yellow in both cases.

Place a large iron pot on the fire. Add vegetable oil. When hot, add chicken wings and brown slightly. Add the turmeric coconut milk. Add all other ingredients except the whole peppers. If there is not enough coconut milk to cover these, add a little water or normal milk. Add the whole peppers, tied in muslin cloth in case they break. Cover until mixture begins to boil.

Meanwhile, in a bowl, begin the dumplings by mixing the flour and butter. Crumble the mixture. Add the salt and cinnamon and mix well. Add enough water to make a sticky but firm dough, form the dough into small balls, roll into 4-inch lengths, and set aside.

Allow the oil-down to slowly boil for approximately 45 minutes, adding the dumplings 20 minutes before it is finished, while there is still liquid. Cover for 5 minutes. Remove cover, stirring now to ensure that the bottom of the oil-down does not begin to burn. When finished and all ingredients are cooked but not mushy, serve in calabash bowls (or ceramic bowls) and eat with a spoon. The pepper can now be removed from the muslin cloth and mashed, and a little can be placed on the oil-down for those who can tolerate the pepper. Salt and pepper can be added to taste.

Further Reading

Parkinson, Rosemary. *Culinaria: The Caribbean*. Cologne, Germany: Könemann, 1999.

Wilkinson, Wendy, and Lee Wilkinson. *Morgan Freeman and Friends: Caribbean Cooking for a Cause*. Emmaus, PA: Rodale Books, 2006.

Guatemala

Population: 14,373,472 (July 2013 est.)
Population Rank: 69th
Population Growth Rate: 1.91% (2013 est.)
Life Expectancy at Birth: 71.46 years (2013 est.)
Health Expenditures: 6.7% of GDP (2011)
People with Access to Safe Drinking Water: 92% of population (2010 est.)

Average Daily Caloric Consumption: 2,170
Adult Obesity Rate: 19.2% (2008)
Underweight Children under Age 5: 13% (2009)

Healthy communities in Guatemala are tied both physically and metaphori-
cally to healthy maize harvests. For thousands of years, Maya households
have blessed a single ear of corn, which is neither planted nor eaten for the
entire season, at the beginning of the harvest. To this day, corn is a symbol
of life and health, and many families continue to practice the ancient birthing
ritual of cutting the umbilical cord above an ear of corn. Contemporary Maya
shamans make use of carefully guarded herbal recipes employed for both religious and medicinal purposes.

Today, lack of access to clean water severely compromises good health for
many Guatemalans. While Guatemala's traditional staple foods are the core
of a healthy diet (beans combined with maize to make up a complete protein,
a diversity of vitamin-rich vegetables, little meat, and many dishes prepared
without animal fat of any kind), struggles related to diet in Guatemala and

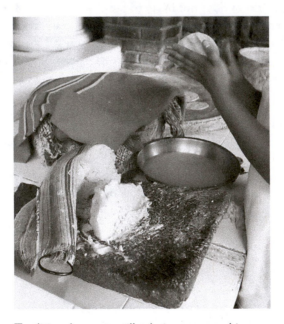

Traditional corn tortillas being prepared in
Guatemala. (Steve Burger/iStockphoto.com)

throughout Central American include diabetes provoked and agitated by increased consumption of processed foods and rampant malnutrition as a consequence of extreme poverty.

Emily Stone

Further Reading

Coe, Sophie D., and Michael D. Coe. *The True History of Chocolate*. 2nd ed. New York: Thames and Hudson, 2007.

McDonald, Michael R. *Food Culture in Central America*. Westport, CT: Greenwood Press, 2009.

Guyana

Population: 739,903 (July 2013 est.)
Population Rank: 164th
Population Growth Rate: –0.21% (2013 est.)
Life Expectancy at Birth: 67.68 years (2013 est.)
Health Expenditures: 5.9% of GDP (2011)
People with Access to Safe Drinking Water: 94% of population (2010 est.)
Average Daily Caloric Consumption: 2,750
Adult Obesity Rate: 17.2% (2008)
Underweight Children under Age 5: 11.1% (2009)

The Guyanese diet is full of a variety of foods, but the goal is to maintain a healthy, balanced diet, which can be difficult, particularly in rural areas. With a poor economy, relying too heavily on inexpensive and plentiful ground provisions may mean missing out on important nutrients, which could lead to malnutrition, especially among children. The Food and Nutrition Unit of Guyana's Ministry of Health is working hard toward making sure the country's citizens have access to and maintain a healthy diet.

Erin Laverty

Further Reading

Houston, Lynn Marie. *Food Culture in the Caribbean*. Westport, CT: Greenwood Press, 2005.

Narine, Nirmala. *In Nirmala's Kitchen: Everyday World Cuisine*. New York: Lake Isle Press, 2006.

Haiti

Population: 9,893,934 (July 2013 est.)
Population Rank: 88th
Population Growth Rate: 0.99% (2013 est.)
Life Expectancy at Birth: 62.85 years (2013 est.)
Health Expenditures: 7.9% of GDP (2011)
People with Access to Safe Drinking Water: 69% of population (2010 est.)
Average Daily Caloric Consumption: 1,850
Adult Obesity Rate: 7.9% (2008)
Underweight Children under Age 5: 18.9% (2006)

Aside from some of the foods associated with vodun, Haitians profess beliefs about food as it relates to health. In Haiti, bread soup is said to have properties similar to those of chicken soup in U.S. culture. Pineapple-skin juice is thought to be a blood and body cleanser, while people believe that drinking beet juice will rejuvenate and invigorate people, by putting more red in their blood, and give them strength for difficult and trying times.

Humoral medical theories, based on ancient Greek ideas passed down through the centuries by groups throughout the Mediterranean, still hold sway in Haiti, particularly in rural areas. Many people in rural Haiti suffer from varying degrees of malnutrition. Hot-cold beliefs impact greatly on nutritional status, particularly that of pregnant and lactating women. One practice illustrating the poverty of Haiti is the eating of clay by pregnant women, which may increase their calcium intake, a practice also common in parts of Africa.

Mudcakes, called *teh*, are eaten in conditions of extreme hunger. People take what vegetables they can find and mix these with mud that has been strained to get out the stones and other debris. They form the mud and vegetables into flat cakes and then dry them in the sun. People eat them like that, without further cooking or preparation. In contrast, obesity is becoming a problem among those Haitians with more money to spend on food.

Cynthia D. Bertelsen

Further Reading

Houston, Lynn Marie. *Food Culture in the Caribbean*. Westport, CT: Greenwood Press, 2005.

Yurnet-Thomas, Mirta. *A Taste of Haiti*. Exp. ed. New York: Hippocrene Books, 2007.

Honduras

Population: 8,448,465 (July 2013 est.)
Population Rank: 93rd
Population Growth Rate: 1.79% (2013 est.)
Life Expectancy at Birth: 70.81 years (2013 est.)
Health Expenditures: 9.1% of GDP (2009)
People with Access to Safe Drinking Water: 87% of population
    (2010 est.)
Average Daily Caloric Consumption: 2,600
Adult Obesity Rate: 18.4% (2008)
Underweight Children under Age 5: 8.6% (2006)

As is the case in many cultures, Hondurans associate various foods and dishes with good health and with cures for sick people. Some of these beliefs include the idea that meat tenderizers like papaya cause stomach ulcers. Sick people, including those with ulcers, should eat *leche dormida* ("sleeping milk"), made with part of a rennet tablet and sweetened to taste, resulting in a dish very similar to yogurt. Many old beliefs—such as the old hot-cold theory—no longer hold, but some people still drink sour orange juice when they do not feel well to balance out their systems. Drinking lemongrass tea for nerve problems is still common in some areas. Folk belief has it that drinking a tea made from *kalaica*, a plant that grows wild in Honduras, will help anemia, as will drinking an infusion made with beets. Many beliefs surround the states of pregnancy and lactation, including the exclusion of certain foods from the diets of pregnant and lactating mothers.

In Honduras, people still experience severe malnutrition, particularly children. One out of four Honduran children under the age of five still suffers from life-threatening bouts of malnutrition, exacerbated by diseases like chickenpox and measles.

Cynthia D. Bertelsen

Further Reading

Gold, Janet N. *Culture and Customs of Honduras.* Santa Barbara, CA: Greenwood Press, 2009.

McDonald, Michael R. *Food Culture in Central America.* Westport, CT: Greenwood Press, 2009.

Inuit

Increased modernization and the availability of *qallunaat*, or white people's food, has had an impact on the health of the Inuit. The shift from the traditional diet of meat and fish to a diet of processed foods high in sugar and carbohydrates has caused an increase in obesity, cardiovascular disease, acne, anemia, dental cavities, and type 2 diabetes. To try and understand the paradox of the Inuit diet—the fact that eating a diet of seal meat, which is high in fat, prevents the very diseases that are common throughout much of the Western world—researchers at McGill University's Centre for Indigenous Peoples' Nutrition and Environment have carefully documented the traditional foods eaten by Inuit peoples, complete with a nutritional and caloric analysis of each of the different Inuit foods.

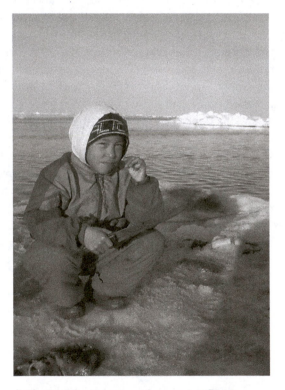

An Inuit girl eats raw seal on an ice floe in Nunavut, Canada. (Paul Nicklen/National Geographic/Getty Images)

What has been discovered is that there are no essential foods, only essential nutrients. And the Inuit get these nutrients in their traditional diet. Vitamin A, for example, which is usually found in fruits and vegetables, is available to the Inuit in the oils of cold-water fish and sea mammals, as well as in the animals' livers, where fat is processed. These dietary staples also provide vitamin D, another oil-soluble vitamin needed for bones. Vitamin C is found in raw caribou liver, seal brains, and maktaaq, and in even higher levels in kelp. The traditional Inuit practices of freezing meat and fish and eating them raw conserve the vitamins, which are easily cooked off and lost in food processing.

The Inuit are genetically well adapted to process a diet that is high in protein. However, protein cannot be the sole source of energy for humans; anyone eating a high-protein diet that is low in carbohydrates must also have fat. While fats are considered to be detrimental to Western health, it is the kind of fat that is eaten that is important. Processed and farm animal fat is high in trans fats, whereas wild animal fat is healthier because it is less saturated and more of it is in a monounsaturated form. In addition, the traditional Inuit diet consists of cold-water fish and sea mammals that are high in omega-3 fats, while a Western diet is high in omega-6 fats. Omega-3 fats help raise high-density lipoprotein (HDL) cholesterol, lower triglycerides, and are known for anticlotting effects. These fatty acids are believed to protect the heart from life-threatening arrhythmias that can lead to sudden cardiac death. In addition, omega-3 polyunsaturated fats help prevent inflammatory processes, which play a part in atherosclerosis, arthritis, diabetes, and other diseases commonly associated with a Western diet.

While the positive aspects of eating traditional Inuit food have been accepted, data also show that there is an increase in the levels of cadmium, lead, and mercury in the traditional meat and fish eaten by the Inuit. Increased levels of PCBs (polychlorinated biphenyls) and DDT (dichlorodiphenyltrichloroethane) have also been found in traditional Inuit foods. The ingestion of metals and chemicals has been found to affect the neurological development of fetuses and children and can affect the immune systems of children. The primary foods that account for a higher level of intake of metals and chemicals are ringed seal meat and liver, caribou meat, narwhal maktaaq, beluga meat, and beluga maktaaq.

Despite the potential dangers of eating country food, the Inuit remain strongly tied to their traditional diet. For the Inuit the connection between eating seal and Inuit beliefs about health, physiology, and identity is stronger than the fears associated with the contaminants found in Arctic foods, and thus country food remains the main diet choice for Inuit today. The traditional

Inuit diet is more nutritious and less expensive than commercial food, and it is believed to have healing properties. If an Inuit is feeling well, then he can eat store-bought food with no ill effects, but if he is ill or depressed, he needs country food to make him well. The Inuit believe strongly that their diet of seal meat is life giving. Inuit blood is believed to be thick and dark like seal blood, so when one eats seal blood and seal meat, one is rejuvenating one's blood supply. Eating seal meat, they believe, warms them in the cold Arctic weather, and when the body is warmed by seal blood, then the Inuit's soul is protected from illness and harm.

Laura P. Appell-Warren

Further Reading

Collings, Peter, George Wenzel, and Richard G. Condon. "Modern Food Sharing Networks and Community Integration in the Central Canadian Arctic." *Arctic* 51, No. 4 (1998): 301–14.

Condon, Richard G. *The Northern Copper Inuit: A History.* Toronto: University of Toronto Press, 1996.

Kuhnlein, Harriet, Oliver Receveur, and Amy Ing. "Energy, Fat and Calcium in Bannock Consumed by Canadian Inuit." *Journal of the American Dietetic Association* 101, No. 5 (2001): 580–81.

Jamaica

Population: 2,909,714 (July 2013 est.)
Population Rank: 139th
Population Growth Rate: 0.7% (2013 est.)
Life Expectancy at Birth: 73.44 years (2013 est.)
Health Expenditures: 5.2% of GDP (2010)
People with Access to Safe Drinking Water: 93% of population (2010 est.)
Average Daily Caloric Consumption: 2,850
Adult Obesity Rate: 24.1% (2008)
Underweight Children under Age 5: 1.9% (2007)

Various medical and belief systems from the indigenous Arawak Indians, African slaves, and Europeans, primarily Spanish and British, have influenced the contemporary Jamaican folk medical system. Indigenous people developed knowledge of medicinal herbs that were available on the island. The Europeans brought the Hippocratic humoral system, based on the idea that the body is regulated by four fluids, blood, phlegm, black bile, and yellow bile, each of which is described as being hot or cold and wet or dry.

During the slavery era, slaves adapted and utilized the concept of obeah, a morally neutral spiritual power, folk magic, or sorcery, which was derived from Central and West African origins. Later, obeah practitioners, yard healers, and bush doctors or herbalists, who normally combine their spiritual and herbal knowledge, became primary healers during the postemancipation era.

Today, most Jamaicans employ both Western biomedical and folk medical systems. Jamaicans attempt to treat an illness first at home using their herbal knowledge or with help from herbalists or bush doctors. Some herbs are linked to the supernatural roles they play in healing. A number of herbs that have been recognized as medicinal are available in Jamaica. "Duppy" (spirit) coconut, "duppy cherry," and "duppy cotton" are some examples of herbs that are related to spirits. If the home remedy is not effective, Jamaicans go to the biomedical doctor that practices Western medicine. If this does not work, some of them ask spiritual practitioners for help or use both biomedical and folk medicine concurrently. Physicians and patients often have different concepts about causes of illness, symptoms, treatment, and lifestyle factors such as diet, which often creates miscommunication.

Besides the use of plants to prevent or treat illnesses, Jamaicans perceive that diet is associated with their health. The Rastafarians are a group of people who generally follow strict guidelines regarding diet. Eating pork and crustaceans is universally prohibited among Rastas. They also tend to be vegetarians and avoid eating other meats such as beef, chicken, and goat. Many Rastas also avoid consuming fish with no scales or large fish, which are perceived to have more developed souls. Most Rastas believe in not killing other creatures and, therefore, prefer a vegan lifestyle, which is referred to as ital, meaning a natural and healthy way of life. Because of their adherence to nature and their belief that their bodies are the temple of the living God, most Rastas also avoid processed foods, which are not ital and pollute their bodies. The use of any added salt is discouraged among Rastafarians.

Because Rastafarians believe in nature's magical healing properties, they rely on herbs and trees instead of pharmaceuticals. Religious healers called Rasta doctors practice in their "balm" yard, an herbal healing garden where the doctors practice their magic, utilizing different herbs as nature (herbs) provides remedy to any illness.

Obesity has become a major public health issue in many developed and developing countries including Jamaica. Diet has been identified as a major factor associated with onset of obesity in those countries. Recent studies have demonstrated that increased fiber intakes in women, as well as increased vegetable consumption in both genders, were associated with a lower body mass index, indicating that promoting a traditional food culture that emphasizes the consumption of fiber-rich vegetables, fruits, and grains may be important to prevent obesity and noncommunicable diseases in Jamaica. At the same time, child undernutrition, especially stunting, is still a public health issue in Jamaica. Researchers in Jamaica recently revealed that stunting was associated with poor psychological functioning in late adolescence. Just like other middle-income countries, Jamaica is experiencing the coexistence of under- and overnutrition, and globalization and lifestyle changes appear to play an important role in Jamaica's nutrition transition.

Keiko Goto

Easter Spice Bun

2 c brown sugar
1 beaten egg
1 tbsp butter
¾ c whole milk
3 tsp baking powder
1 tsp grated nutmeg
1 tsp cinnamon
Pinch of salt
1 tbsp vanilla
1 c raisins
½ tsp lime juice

Grease a loaf tin and line it with greased paper.
Preheat oven to 350°F for about 15 minutes.
Add sugar to beaten egg, and then add melted butter and milk.
Add all dry ingredients, and beat until smooth.
Add vanilla and the fresh raisins to the mix, plus lime juice, and then pour into the lined and greased tin.
Bake for approximately 1 hour.

Glaze
½ c brown sugar
½ c water

Boil water and sugar until thick.

Spread the glaze on the Easter bun, and return to the oven for an additional 5–8 minutes.

If desired, press a few whole cherries into the top of the bun.

Further Reading

Higman, B. W. *Jamaican Food: History, Biology, Culture*. Kingston, Jamaica: University of West Indies Press, 2008.

Higman, B.W. "Jamaican Versions of Callaloo." *Callaloo* 30, No. 1 (2007): 351–68.

Houston, Lynn Marie. *Food Culture in the Caribbean*. Westport, CT: Greenwood Press, 2005.

Martinique and Guadeloupe

For French citizens residing in the overseas departments of Martinique, Guadeloupe, and French Guiana, life expectancy has continued to rise during the 2000s so that it now matches that of metropolitan France: 81 years as of 2013. This rise in life expectancy is almost entirely due to a decrease in infant mortality. In terms of health, high blood pressure, cancer, and cardiovascular disease are the most important threats to life expectancy on the islands, as they are in metropolitan France and in the West, generally. One enormous difference in the health of metropolitan and overseas French citizens is caused by endocrinal diseases, which kill at double the rate on Guadeloupe, Martinique, and French Guiana compared to the metropole. All of these pathologies are linked to diet, and endocrinal disease in particular is connected to type 2 or sugar diabetes, which can develop in those whose diets feature too much starchy and sweet food. Diabetes affects women in the overseas departments at a higher rate than men.

The rates and nature of alcohol-related problems also differ between the metropole and the islands. While alcoholic psychosis kills at a higher rate overseas, cirrhosis of the liver kills at a lower rate, with Guadeloupe being the island most affected by all alcoholic disorders. The reason for this discrepancy lies in the type of alcohol consumed: rum on the islands and wine in the metropole. These statistics notwithstanding, female alcoholism is lower on Martinique and French Guiana than in the metropole.

While health is assessed and medical care is provided on the islands in institutionally similar ways to metropolitan France, there exists nonetheless in the French Antilles an extensive body of folk remedies that rely on local plants for the production of botanical tonics (*rimèd razié*). Considered part of the legacy of slaves' knowledge of healing, this body of knowledge is currently experiencing a renewal of interest. On Guadeloupe, for example, the Association pour la promotion et le développement des plantes médicinales et aromatiques de Guadeloupe (Association for the Promotion and Development of Medicinal and Aromatic Plants of Guadeloupe) has inventoried 625 varieties of medicinal plants that can be used to create remedies. While some of these remedies are familiar to all localities where the particular plant grows—for instance, using cloves to soothe toothaches—there are many specific to the islands. Examples include a flower called *atoumo* in Creole ("against all evils"), whose petals in combination with rum and honey are considered to bring down fevers; the bark of the red gum tree (*gommier rouge*) macerated with allspice berries in rum, which is thought to soothe rheumatism; and a bath containing the leaves of the sugar apple (*pomme cannelle*), which is reported to lift fatigue.

Bertie Mandelblatt

Further Reading

Burton, David. *French Colonial Cookery: A Cook's Tour of the French-Speaking World*. London: Faber and Faber, 2000.

De Rozières, Babette. *Creole: Recipes from the Culinary Heritage of the Caribbean, Blending Asian, African, Indian, and European Traditions*. London: Phaidon, 2007.

Ovide, Stéphanie. *French Caribbean Cuisine*. New York: Hippocrene Books, 2002.

Mexico

Population: 116,220,947 (July 2013 est.)
Population Rank: 11th
Population Growth Rate: 1.07% (2013 est.)
Life Expectancy at Birth: 76.86 years (2013 est.)
Health Expenditures: 6.4% of GDP (2009)
People with Access to Safe Drinking Water: 96% of population (2010 est.)
Average Daily Caloric Consumption: 3,250
Adult Obesity Rate: 32.1% (2008)
Underweight Children under Age 5: 3.4% (2006)

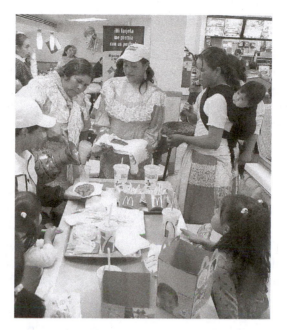

Women offer traditional tortillas and Mexican sauces to patrons of a McDonald's in the Mexican city of Toluca. (Mario Vazquez/AFP/ Getty Images)

Mexico is a country of profound and often conflicting contrasts. At the same time as government and health officials attempt to cope with malnutrition and anemia in rural Mexico, one in every three adults in urban Mexico is overweight, making obesity the most serious health problem in the country today. The problems of malnutrition and anemia are proving to be easier to resolve than obesity, which has risen to epidemic levels during the past decade.

Mexican food habits have changed substantially in the past few years. Nutritionists have observed an increase in the consumption of wheat products, replacing corn, in the form of breads, cereals, pastas, cookies, and pastries. This is in part caused by the transition from a rural to an urban diet due to the heavy migration from the countryside to urban areas during the past few decades. The general availability of refined, high-fat, and high-sugar products in urban areas makes fast-food products convenient purchases.

The new products available on the market, introduced by the North American Free Trade Agreement in 1994, often replace rather than complement Mexican ingredients in the diet. The increased participation of women in the labor force results in less time for women to prepare family meals and forces them to rely on ready-made foods, which may be higher in fats and simple carbohydrates than homemade meals. There is also a tendency to accept the new food imports because of their higher status compared to the traditional diet, especially for those at middle and high income levels. The external influence is less dramatic on rural diets; however, the migration of undocumented Mexican laborers to the United States has proved detrimental to the rural diet as well, when workers return with a preference for diets high in animal fats and sugars. The frequency of obesity, diabetes, and cardiovascular problems as a result of the change to a more refined diet high in fats and sugars can be observed in both urban as well as rural Mexico.

For several decades, the Mexican government has carried out various programs in an attempt to improve the diet and nutrition of the Mexican population. These have included changes in economic policies, control of food prices, subsidies for the production of food, retail sale of government-subsidized foods, and programs of food distribution. These include free primary-school breakfasts in rural schools and food boxes or baskets containing products that make up the basic diet.

One of the most noted deficiencies in the Mexican diet at all social levels is iron, which reflects an inadequate diet. This has been shown to cause anemia in both children and expectant mothers, as well as retarded growth patterns in children. School-age children who are affected by an iron deficiency show less interest in learning, a reduced attention span, and chronic fatigue. Anemia is more prevalent in rural Mexico than in urban communities.

Nutrients have been added to industrialized food products in the form of vitamins and minerals since 1987 in an effort to improve the Mexican diet. The addition of vitamins and minerals to both wheat and corn flour plays an important role in the Mexican diet, as many products are made from these basic ingredients.

Obesity represents the most serious health problem in Mexico today. One in every three urban adults in Mexico is overweight or obese, and the prediction is for these numbers to continue rising for both children and adults in coming years. The increase in excessive weight and obesity is associated with chronic diseases such as type 2 diabetes mellitus, hypertension, atherosclerosis, high cholesterol, certain types of cancer, cardiovascular diseases, and orthopedic, respiratory, and psychological problems. Coping with the health costs that result from obesity is a heavy burden for the Mexican health system to carry. Thirty percent of obesity is attributed to cultural factors, such as the high-fat diet popular in Mexico and a general lack of discipline in food habits. Soft drinks, such as Coca-Cola and Pepsi, contribute heavily to obesity, because Mexicans drink on average more than a 12-ounce can of soda every day. Forty-five percent of the cases of obesity are attributed to nontransmissible environmental factors. The consumption of processed foods with a high oil content and of simple and refined carbohydrates, with less fiber and complex carbohydrates, plays a role in the surge in obesity.

Recent statistics indicate that 10.75 percent of Mexicans between the ages of 20 and 69 are afflicted by some type of diabetes mellitus, which is equivalent to more than 5.5 million persons. Almost 23 percent of those affected with diabetes are unaware they have the illness. It is one of the principal causes of death in Mexico, along with cardiovascular problems and cancer. Obesity has become one of the major factors in the risk of acquiring the disease. A diet high in carbohydrates, lack of exercise, excess weight, chronic stress, and inheritance all play a role in the disease.

Anorexia is a growing problem in Mexico and has increased considerably in the past five years. It is more prevalent among young women than in young men and affects mostly young people between the ages of 11 and 25. Food deprivation is not a novelty in Mexico. It was common behavior in Catholic convents, where food was considered a spiritual element that converted eating into a ritual act. The convent dining room was a space of penitence and purification, where food was transformed into something sacred through which the nuns could expunge their sins and purify their spirits. Fasting and penitence were methods by which they attempted to attain purification of their bodies and souls. To leave a morsel of their favorite dish on their plate for the guardian angel was considered a manifestation of high spirituality.

Janet Long-Solís

Further Reading

Long, J., ed. *Conquista y Comida: Consecuencias del encuentro de dos mundos.* Mexico City: Universidad Nacional Autónoma de México, 1996.

Long-Solís, Janet. *Food Culture in Mexico.* Westport, CT: Greenwood Press, 2005.

Pilcher, J. *¡Que vivan los tamales! Food and the Making of Mexican Identity.* Albuquerque: University of New Mexico Press, 1998.

Native Americans

Many of the most common causes of death among Native Americans are directly related to diet. Many medical and nutrition experts agree that the radical changes in Native diets due to displacement to reservations have had a direct effect on the physical health of this population. Heart disease is the leading cause of death among Native Americans, and diet-related obesity, high blood pressure, high cholesterol, and diabetes are all risk factors associated with heart disease. Experts indicate that, on average, 30 percent of Native adults are obese. In some areas, like Arizona, nearly 95 percent of Native diabetics are also overweight.

Fry bread is often scapegoated as a primary cause for obesity and diabetes in Native populations. Because it is fried bread drenched in grease, it has nearly no nutritional value and is ultimately a delivery mechanism for 25 grams of excess fat and 700 empty calories (U.S. Department of Agriculture). Fry bread, along with other government-supplied commodity foods like potted meats, lard, and processed cheese, is often blamed for the widespread obesity and diabetes "epidemic" among Native populations. Many Native activists feel that these problems are a direct result of government programs of relocating tribes to reservations, thereby cutting them off from their traditional lifestyles, which lent the Native American diet a natural form of regulated caloric intake, an optimal balance of nutrients, and survival-inspired dietary adaptations.

In addition to having extremely high-fat diets and sedentary lifestyles, malnutrition is also a problem among Native American peoples; studies show that a mere 21 percent eat the recommended amount of fruit on any given day, while 34 percent eat the recommended amount of vegetables. The extreme poverty of reservation life also leads to prevalent hunger: Native Americans are also four times more likely to report not having enough to eat than other U.S. households. Proper nutrition education would help to mitigate this problem.

Other, more obscure threats to Native diets present themselves in genetically modified organisms (GMOs). While naturally growing wild rice crops in Wisconsin and Minnesota have dwindled to half in the past century, agricultural firms and food corporations have developed a way to grow cultivated or paddy "wild" rice, which poses a threat to the Ojibwe, who rely on proper wild rice for income and preservation of their culture and traditions. There is fear among the Ojibwe that genetically modified rice may come to contaminate the naturally occurring wild rice they depend on; residents of the White Earth reservation in Minnesota have launched the Save Wild Rice campaign to prevent this from happening.

Melanie Haupt

Fry Bread

Makes 6–8 large fry breads

3 c all-purpose flour
1 tbsp baking powder
1 tsp salt
1 1/4 c warm water
Extra flour for processing
Vegetable oil for frying, or lard (traditional)

Blend the flour with the baking powder and salt in a mixing bowl. Make a well in the center of the flour mixture, and pour in the warm water. Mix the flour and water with a wooden spoon. Take the dough from the bowl, and mix gently with hands on a board until dough is thoroughly mixed. Excessive kneading will make a heavy fry bread. Form into a ball. Cover dough with a kitchen towel, and let rest for 10 minutes. Place dough on a cutting board, and cut dough into 6–8 pieces. Shape and pat each piece into a disk 5–7 inches in diameter.

Place vegetable oil or lard in deep, heavy pan. Oil should be a minimum of 1 inch deep. Heat oil to about 350°F. Place formed dough gently in oil, and press down on dough as it fries so the top is submerged in the hot oil. Do not overcrowd pan. Fry until some browning occurs, approximately 2–3 minutes, then flip and fry other side. Bread is done when surface is dry to the touch and smooth.

Further Reading

Berzok, Linda Murray. *American Indian Food*. Westport, CT: Greenwood Press, 2005.

Divina, Fernando. *Foods of the Americas: Native Recipes and Traditions*. Berkeley, CA: Ten Speed Press, 2004.

Mihesuah, Devon A. *Recovering Our Ancestors' Gardens: Indigenous Recipes and Guide to Diet and Fitness*. Lincoln: University of Nebraska Press, 2005.

Nicaragua

Population: 5,788,531 (July 2013 est.)
Population Rank: 109th
Population Growth Rate: 1.05% (2013 est.)
Life Expectancy at Birth: 72.45 years (2013 est.)
Health Expenditures: 10.1% of GDP (2009)
People with Access to Safe Drinking Water: 85% of population (2010 est.)
Average Daily Caloric Consumption: 2,400
Adult Obesity Rate: 22.2% (2008)
Underweight Children under Age 5: 5.7% (2007)

Poverty is the main social determinant of the quality of diet and overall health status in Nicaragua, and the traditional diet has undergone a transition, fueled by globalization and urbanization. Major changes in trade and exchange among nation-states have meant for people on the ground an increased use of processed foods including sugar, refined flour, hydrogenated fats, and animal products coupled with a decline in the intake of whole grains, fruit, and vegetables of local provenance. Despite the availability of many healthful foods, the average Nicaraguan's diet is unbalanced. Various data concur that more than a fifth of the overall population is malnourished, and approximately one in four children in Nicaragua is stunted due to malnutrition. Paradoxically, Nicaragua has witnessed a growing incidence of obesity, diabetes, and cardiovascular disease in the same era. A health problem related to diet is the lack of access to sanitation and safe drinking water. Most rural dwellers in Nicaragua rely on contaminated water sources, and a significant proportion of the overall population does not have access to basic sanitation. Both factors amplify various health problems originating in poor diet.

Good health in Nicaragua is challenged by a wide array of health problems including a high prevalence of malaria and other parasitic diseases, various respiratory ailments, diarrheal diseases, anemia, periodic natural disasters, malnutrition, and high rates of maternal and infant mortality. The Sandinista regime substantially increased spending on health care, broadening and equalizing access to services. There was a substantial drop in infant mortality and the transmission of communicable diseases. However, the system was increasingly strained by shortages of funds. The current health care system aligned against these challenges mirrors the stratified nature of Nicaraguan society. Members of the upper classes rely on private physicians and hospitals, and often travel abroad for specialized care. The Nicaraguan Social

Security Institute provides health care to the small segment of society employed in government and industry. The vast majority of the population is served at public facilities, and some 40 percent of Nicaraguans have no access to any health care services due to the uneven provision of services and the locations of health care facilities.

Various governmental and nongovernmental programs have taken aim at overall health status by improving people's food security and nutritional health. For instance, a program of free school meals for all primary-school children provides daily meals of rice, beans, corn, oil, and cereal, which are prepared by parents in rotation as part of a school-supervised food-aid program. Likewise, the government has distributed food-production packages including livestock, seeds, and agricultural inputs to families in rural areas of Nicaragua to boost food production and stabilize rural communities.

Michael R. McDonald

Pinolillo

3 ears fresh maize on the cob
$1/2$ c cocoa powder
$1/2$ tsp cinnamon
$1/2$ tsp salt
2 tsp ancho chili powder
Sugar to taste

Remove husks and silk from maize, and boil ears of maize for approximately 12 minutes or microwave at high heat for 6 minutes (long enough to allow the kernels to be removed from the cob easily). Remove kernels from cobs and spread on a baking sheet; sprinkle lightly with salt and place in a 325°F oven for approximately 10 minutes, or until the kernels appear lightly toasted. Monitor closely to guard against burning.

Place all ingredients into a blender or food processor, and blend on low speed for about a minute or until the corn kernels are pulverized.

Pour mixture over ice or add to $1/2$ glass of cold milk, and sweeten to taste.

Further Reading

Behnke, Alison, Griselda Aracely Chacon, and Kristina Anderson. *Cooking the Central American Way: Culturally Authentic Foods, Including Low-Fat and Vegetarian Recipes.* Minneapolis, MN: Lerner, 2005.

McDonald, Michael R. *Food Culture in Central America*. Westport, CT: Greenwood Press, 2009.

White, Stephen F., and Esthela Calderon. *Culture and Customs of Nicaragua*. Westport, CT: Greenwood Press, 2008.

Panama

Population: 3,559,408 (July 2013 est.)
Population Rank: 131st
Population Growth Rate: 1.38% (2013 est.)
Life Expectancy at Birth: 78.13 years (2013 est.)
Health Expenditures: 8.2% of GDP (2011)
People with Access to Safe Drinking Water: 93% of population (2008 est.)
Average Daily Caloric Consumption: 2,450
Adult Obesity Rate: 25.4% (2008)
Underweight Children under Age 5: 3.9% (2008)

Studies conducted in connection to the dietary practices of Panamanians indicate that excess consumption of oil and salt among most ethnic groups has produced frequent cases of hypertension and obesity, in both urban and rural areas. Exceptions include the diets considered traditional for rural populations and indigenous peoples, such as the Kuna, whose diet has been studied from nutritional and cultural perspectives recently. The Kuna who have moved to urban areas and away from their *comarcas* (administrative regions with substantial indigenous populations) have tended to adapt to the less healthy dietary norms of mainstream Panama. A similar situation occurs with the largest indigenous group in Panama, the Ngöbe. Among the Ngöbe, greater involvement in the cash economy and greater availability of cash, due to government subsidies and more people working for wages, have produced a substantial shift away from the traditional diet, which was nutritionally balanced overall. The Ngöbe diet now includes large quantities of purchased polished white rice and white sugar and less of the traditional healthy foods. Consequently, rates of undernutrition and malnutrition have risen substantially.

Carla Guerrón Montero

Further Reading
McDonald, Michael R. *Food Culture in Central America*. Santa Barbara, CA: Greenwood Press/ABC-Clio, 2009.

Williams, Chuck, ed. *Essentials of Latin Cooking*. Birmingham, AL: Oxmoor House, 2010.

Paraguay and Uruguay

Paraguay

Population: 6,623,252 (July 2013 est.)
Population Rank: 103rd
Population Growth Rate: 1.23% (2013 est.)
Life Expectancy at Birth: 76.6 years (2013 est.)
Health Expenditures: 9.7% of GDP (2011)
People with Access to Safe Drinking Water: 86% of population (2010 est.)
Average Daily Caloric Consumption: 2,620
Adult Obesity Rate: 17.9% (2008)
Underweight Children under Age 5: 3.4% (2005)

Uruguay

Population: 3,324,460 (July 2013 est.)
Population Rank: 134th
Population Growth Rate: 0.25% (2013 est.)
Life Expectancy at Birth: 76.61 years (2013 est.)
Health Expenditures: 8% of GDP (2011)
People with Access to Safe Drinking Water: 100% of population (2010 est.)
Average Daily Caloric Consumption: 2,820
Adult Obesity Rate: 24.8% (2008)
Underweight Children under Age 5: 6% (2004)

Uruguay has one of the best health systems in South America, and life expectancy is high for the region. The country has one of the lowest poverty levels on the continent, and energy and protein malnutrition are not serious threats. Most of Uruguay's health problems are those associated with excess. Obesity is quite prevalent and is caused by a high consumption of beef and dairy products, which lead to a diet rich in saturated fats. The Uruguayan diet also includes high consumption of sugars and carbohydrates in the form of potatoes, pastas, breads, sodas, alcoholic beverages, and sugary desserts. The major causes of death in Uruguay are diet related and include heart disease, cancer, and digestive disorders. Uruguay has the highest percentage of diabetics in South America. Studies suggest that Uruguayans' knowledge, attitudes, and practices concerning food and nutrition are inadequate, and measures are being taken to influence dietary choices to include more fruits, vegetables, fish, and fiber.

In Paraguay, access to proper health care and fresh drinking water varies greatly from city to countryside. Paraguay also has among the lowest rates of undernourishment and malnutrition in Latin America, yet deficiency disorders do occur, especially among the lowest-income population and in rural areas. The typical Paraguayan diet includes a high amount of carbohydrates and saturated fats. Yucca is the main source of carbohydrates, but corn products, sodas, fruit juices, sugar, and beer also contribute. Saturated fats come in the form of meat, especially beef, and animal fats used in cooking. Due to changing dietary trends and increasing knowledge among some sections of the population, some Paraguayans are changing traditional recipes by substituting vegetable oils for animal fats such as suet or lard. Cardiovascular diseases are among the leading causes of death for Paraguayan adults.

The botanical-medicinal heritage of the indigenous groups of Paraguay has been preserved to some extent, particularly in rural areas. Paraguayans frequently add herbs to the water used to brew tereré to heal minor ailments such as headaches or stomachaches. Certain traditional dishes are also believed to provide specific health and nutritional benefits. An example is *itacurú cué* (tripe soup), believed to restore health to the ill, provide strength to the frail, and increase milk production for women who are nursing.

Cari Sánchez

Further Reading

Kijac, Maria Baez. *The South American Table*. Boston: Harvard Common Press, 2003.

Lovera, José Rafael. *Food Culture in South America*. Westport, CT: Greenwood Press, 2005.

Velilla de Aquino, Josefina. *Tembi'u Paraguái: Comida paraguaya*. 13th ed. Asunción, Paraguay: RP Ediciones, 2002.

Peru

Population: 29,849,303 (July 2013 est.)
Population Rank: 42nd
Population Growth Rate: 1% (2013 est.)
Life Expectancy at Birth: 72.98 years (2013 est.)
Health Expenditures: 4.8% of GDP (2011)

People with Access to Safe Drinking Water: 85% of population (2010 est.)
Average Daily Caloric Consumption: 2,430
Adult Obesity Rate: 15.7% (2008)
Underweight Children under Age 5: 4.5% (2008)

Archaeological remains of preconquest indigenous Peruvians indicate that they were in good health. Protein sources included cuy (Peruvian guinea pig), game, fish, and quinoa. Dried foods and multiclimatic agricultural practices ensured food security. Moreover, recent analysis of the preconquest indigenous diet reveals that ingestion patterns increased nutrient absorption. The "appetizer" for the midday meal was *cancha* (dried maize). The rough texture of this foodstuff opened the alimentary passages, preparing them for increased nutrient absorption. Custom prevented the drinking of chicha de jora (maize beer) until the end of the meal, when enzymes in this fermented beverage could aid in the digestion of the complex carbohydrate–rich menu. This eliminated the danger of losing nutrients due to excess liquid or fiber pushing food through the digestive system too quickly.

Indigenous Peruvians have chewed the leaves of the coca plant, which are used to make the narcotic drug cocaine, for centuries. When the leaves are chewed alone, they produce a mild burst of energy. When they are chewed with an alkaline agent, usually in the form of vegetal ashes, the effect is heightened. The chewing of coca leaves does not have the extreme narcotic effect of the chemically pure alkaloid cocaine, nor does it seem to be addictive. It seems to help relieve the symptoms of altitude sickness.

Kelly O'Leary

Further Reading

Custer, Tony. *The Art of Peruvian Cuisine*. Lima, Peru: Fundación Custer, 2003.

Kijac, Maria Baez. *The South American Table*. Cambridge, MA: Harvard Common Press, 2003.

Lovera, José Rafael. *Food Culture in South America*. Westport, CT: Greenwood Press, 2005.

Puerto Rico

Population: 3,674,209 (July 2013 est.)
Population Rank: 129th
Population Growth Rate: –0.47% (2013 est.)
Life Expectancy at Birth: 79.07 years (2013 est.)

Health Expenditures: Unknown
People with Access to Safe Drinking Water: Unknown
Average Daily Caloric Consumption: Unknown
Adult Obesity Rate: Unknown
Underweight Children under Age 5: Unknown or Negligible

A history of a plantation economy followed by one dominated by industries and services means that Puerto Rico imports the bulk of its food. There is small-scale production of coffee, bananas, vegetables, poultry, and dairy products, but it is not enough to satisfy local demand, and many local producers find it hard to compete with cheaper food imports. In the twentieth century the Puerto Rican diet shifted from one based on agricultural products and frequent scarcity to one based on agroindustrial processed foods and relative abundance. The results are well known in all industrialized countries: widespread obesity, including high rates of childhood obesity, and related diseases like diabetes, high blood pressure, and heart disease. In 2007 the government of Puerto Rico initiated a campaign to make exercise and nutrition instruction available in all municipalities.

Puerto Ricans are trying to improve the quality of their food in many different ways. Vegetarianism has become established as a viable diet alternative, and many stores and restaurants cater to this lifestyle. There are a few small organic farms, some of which offer community-supported agriculture programs. Most people have switched from lard to olive or vegetable oil, and many try to reduce their consumption of the fried and high-carbohydrate foods that are abundant in the Puerto Rican diet: rice, beans, viandas, fritters. Sedentary lifestyles, an abundance of heavily processed foods, and confusion and misinformation regarding diet and health guidelines are the norm.

Zilkia Janer

Gandules con Bollitos de Plátano
(Pigeon Peas with Green Plantain Dumplings)

Serves 4

For the Bollitos
1 green plantain
1/2 tbsp olive oil
1/2 tsp garlic, crushed
1/4 tsp salt
1/4 tsp ground black pepper

For the Gandules
1 1/2 tbsp olive oil
1 small onion, chopped
1 clove garlic, crushed
2 oz smoked ham, cubed
2 tbsp sofrito (available in the Latin American foods aisle of most supermarkets)
1/4 c tomato sauce
1 can pigeon peas, drained
2 1/2 c water
1 bay leaf
Salt and pepper to taste

Peel the plantain, and grate it using the smallest holes of a box grater. The result should be wet and sticky. Mix the grated plantains with the oil, garlic, salt, and pepper. Take teaspoonfuls of the mixture and shape into small balls. Cover until ready to use.

Heat the oil in a large pot, and sauté the onion, garlic, and ham until the onion is translucent. Add the sofrito, stir, and cook for 3 minutes. Add the tomato sauce, stir, and cook for 3 more minutes. Add the pigeon peas and stir well. Add the water, bay leaf, salt, and pepper, and simmer for 15 minutes. Drop in the dumplings one at a time, and stir carefully after 5 minutes. Simmer for 30 minutes, or until the broth has thickened and the dumplings are cooked through. Serve with white rice.

Further Reading

Benet, Wilo. *Puerto Rico True Flavors*. Baltimore, MD: Read Street, 2007.

Duprey de Sterling, Emma. *Puerto Rican Artisanal Cookery*. San Juan: University of Puerto Rico Press, 2008.

Suriname

Population: 566,846 (July 2013 est.)
Population Rank: 170th
Population Growth Rate: 1.15% (2013 est.)
Life Expectancy at Birth: 71.41 years (2013 est.)
Health Expenditures: 5.3% of GDP (2011)
People with Access to Safe Drinking Water: 92% of population (2010 est.)

Average Daily Caloric Consumption: 2,470
Adult Obesity Rate: 25.1% (2008)
Underweight Children under Age 5: 7.5% (2006)

Despite a wealth of natural resources and a small population of around 500,000, a large number of people in Suriname suffer from malnutrition and a poor health. According to a World Bank Report on Suriname, approximately 47 percent of the population lives in poverty and is deprived of sufficient and healthy nutrition. Although the government is responsible for the promotion, protection, and improvement of public health, Suriname's government lacks funding.

In Suriname, diet and health are intertwined. Hindus, Muslims, Jews, Creoles, and indigenous communities all follow their own medical system, and traditional healers are often consulted. The cuisines of the Chinese Surinamese and Javanese Surinamese communities are considerably healthier than those of the Creole Surinamese and Hindu Surinamese. The Hindu and Creole diets tend to be too fatty and monotonous. Many Creoles follow Winti, a traditional African practice, and largely a secret religion, with its own myths, rites, offerings, spirits, and taboos. In Suriname Winti is influenced by both Christianity and Judaism. In Winti taboos are often related to food and called *treefs* (from the Hebrew *tarefa*, for forbidden food). Similar to in Judaism, for followers of Winti certain types of animal food are prohibited such as turtle and deer but also plants like plantain. Also, *kaseri* (from the Hebrew word *kosher*) plays a role in forbidding, for instance, menstruating women preparing or touching food.

Karin Vaneker

Further Reading

Starke, A. A., and M. Samsin-Hewitt. *Groot Surinaams Kookboek*. Paramaribo, Suriname: Stichting Kakantrie, 1976.

Vaneker, Karin. *Mavis Kookt: De Surinaamse keuken volgens Mavis Hofwijk* [Mavis cooks: Surinamese cuisine according to Mavis Hofwijk]. 's-Gravenland, the Netherlands: Fontaine, 2008.

Trinidad and Tobago

Population: 1,225,225 (July 2013 est.)
Population Rank: 158th
Population Growth Rate: –0.09% (2013 est.)
Life Expectancy at Birth: 71.96 years (2013 est.)

Health Expenditures: 5.7% of GDP (2011)
People with Access to Safe Drinking Water: 94% of population (2010 est.)
Average Daily Caloric Consumption: 2,710
Adult Obesity Rate: 29.3% (2008)
Underweight Children under Age 5: 4.4% (2000)

Trinidadian foods have come to be considered by nutritionists as overly carbohydrate- and fat-rich, based heavily in starches, once used to provide calories to field laborers along with limited protein and poorer, fattier cuts of meat unwanted by plantation masters. Oil, particularly coconut oil, was well used in African, Indian, and Chinese cooking and continues to be so today, even when vegetable or seed oils are substituted. In recent years, the government health department has undertaken health campaigns to promote more judicious use of fats and oils for heart health, as heart disease is the leading cause of disease-related death in Trinidad and Tobago.

According to the United Nations' Food and Agriculture Organization (FAO), obesity is not yet a problem in Trinidad and Tobago among children and young people, much like the United States, though the number of overweight individuals has increased as the country has moved away from an agrarian to an industrial society. The FAO reported in 1999 that nearly 17 percent of people over 20 are overweight, and within that group 31 percent are obese.

Childhood nutrition, particularly regarding the consumption of adequate calcium, is also a concern into which health officials are putting efforts. Hypertension and alcoholism are two other common diet-based health issues. Although no recent data have been gathered about food access, in 1995, 22 percent of the population was listed as living below the poverty level, half of which were considered "extremely poor" and therefore having limited access to food and proper nutrition. Most at risk for malnutrition in those households, according to the FAO, are children, the elderly, and pregnant and lactating women. While Trinidadians do eat a wide variety of fruits and vegetables on a daily basis, they also consume a great deal of sugar as alcohol, and diabetes is on the uptick.

Ramin Ganeshram

Further Reading

Ganeshram, Ramin. *Sweet Hands: Island Cooking from Trinidad and Tobago*. New York: Hippocrene Books, 2006.

Lai, Walton Look. *Indentured Labor, Caribbean Sugar: Chinese and Indian Migrants to the British West Indies, 1838–1918*. Baltimore, MD: Johns Hopkins University Press, 2004.

United States

Population: 316,668,567 (July 2013 est.)
Population Rank: 3rd
Population Growth Rate: 0.9% (2013 est.)
Life Expectancy at Birth: 78.62 years (2013 est.)
Health Expenditures: 17.9% of GDP (2011)
People with Access to Safe Drinking Water: 99% of population (2010 est.)
Average Daily Caloric Consumption: 3,770
Adult Obesity Rate: 33% (2008)
Underweight Children under Age 5: 1.3% (2004)

Hawaii

Prior to Western contact native Hawaiians enjoyed relatively good health. The combination of regular light manual labor and a diet high in nutrients and low in fat was beneficial to the majority of the population. Kalo and 'uala are good sources of vitamins, minerals, and dietary fiber. Native Hawaiians supplemented these starchy foods with fruit, vegetables, and fish. Necessary fats were provided by regular consumption of food such as coconuts and the occasional consumption of pork, dog, and chicken.

Western contact had catastrophic effects on the native Hawaiian population, who had no resistance to the illnesses common to Europe and Asia. Many died in a short period of time, and much was lost. The introduction of new foodways has also been detrimental to native Hawaiians' health. Many new foods, such as white rice, are high in calories and low in nutrients. Eaten in moderation they pose no threat, but these foods have been incorporated into daily life, and Hawaiian portion sizes remain large despite an increasingly sedentary lifestyle. This new diet has led to a number of health problems that continue to plague the native Hawaiian community.

Native Hawaiians are significantly more likely to suffer from obesity, heart disease, and diabetes than members of the other major ethnic groups in Hawaii. These conditions have been directly linked to diet. Native Hawaiians are also more likely to suffer from many forms of cancer, including breast, lung, colon, rectal, and prostate cancer. Native Hawaiians are among the poorest Hawaii residents and some of the most underserviced in terms of health care. They are less likely to receive preventative care, diagnostic care, or treatment than other ethnic groups.

Overall, Hawaii's population is relatively healthy when compared to the rest of the United States. Hawaii has one of the lowest overall rates of adult and childhood obesity. This reflects the active, healthy lifestyle associated with the local culture. Eating patterns in Hawaii are moderate, and dietary excess is offset, in part, by outdoors activities, such as hiking, swimming, and surfing. The obesity rate, however, is following the national trend and increasing. Hawaii's population needs to embrace a healthier diet, but it does not necessarily need to give up tradition to do so.

Kelila Jaffe

Further Reading

Corum, Ann Kondo. *Ethnic Foods of Hawaii.* Honolulu, HI: Bess Press, 2000.

Trubeck, Amy B. *The Taste of Place: A Cultural Journey into Terroir.* Berkeley: University of California Press, 2009.

Yim, Susan. *We Go Eat: A Mixed Plate from Hawaii's Food Culture.* Honolulu: Hawaii Council for the Humanities, 2008.

The Mid-Atlantic

The mid-Atlantic states of the United States are here defined as the heavily urbanized and industrial region stretching from north of Virginia to the south of New England including New York, New Jersey, Pennsylvania, Delaware, and Maryland as well as the interior of these states.

New York City faces the same challenges as the rest of the United States: Obesity/overweight and diabetes are threatening the well-being of large percentages of the population. Obesity, diabetes, and other diet-related diseases are strongly correlated with class, race/ethnicity, and neighborhood. While middle- and upper-income people like Will and Nina live in neighborhoods with many food choices including large grocery stores, specialty stores, restaurants ranging from fast food to full-service, and two farmers' markets within walking distance of their home, too many New Yorkers live in neighborhoods described as "food deserts." Access to fresh, healthy foods is a challenge in these food deserts, and residents are consigned to paying high prices for low-quality foods. Often, they are dependent on bodegas and other small stores with limited selections. Not all vendors accept EBT (food stamps/electronic benefits), WIC coupons, and other forms of social supports, further limiting where people can shop. Compounded with long working hours (many low-income individuals work more than one job), and long routes to and from work, these factors mean shopping is difficult. Kitchens in public housing— let alone shelters and other temporary housing—are often in disrepair. Fast food offers quick satisfaction at a reasonable price—and long-term negative impacts on overall health. A number of recent government initiatives have been established to correct this situation, including federal funds that will help chain groceries build new stores in areas of the Bronx and Brooklyn that have low food access (a program piloted successfully in Philadelphia). GreenCarts is a Department of Health program that issues licenses to pushcart vendors who agree to sell produce in food deserts. Chain restaurants are required to post calorie counts in an effort to help consumers make more informed choices. Trans fats were banned several years ago, causing major food processors to adjust their recipes. The city sent advisors out to bakeries, restaurants, and local manufacturers to help them change their practices. Salt is the new target in an effort to lower rates of hypertension, especially prevalent among lower-income residents. While critics complained that Bill de Blasio was operating a "nanny state," diet-related diseases cost the city millions in health care and lost productivity every year. Without laws that force food processors to institute changes, it is very difficult to address these issues. A large city like New York has the market muscle to make this happen.

New York's Greenmarket program started in 1976 when a farmers' market opened at Union Square to provide farmers within a 200-mile radius of the city with a profitable outlet for their produce, and city residents with fresh fruits and vegetables. Today, Greenmarket operates nearly 50 markets, found in every borough of the city. There are more requests for markets than there

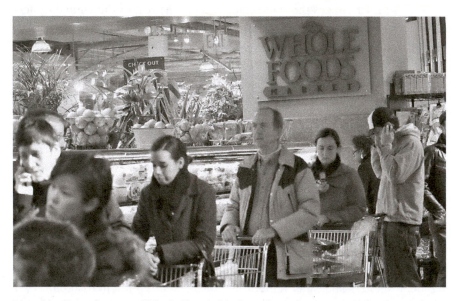

New Yorkers shop at a Whole Foods Market, the largest natural-foods grocer in the United States. (Daniel Acker/Bloomberg/Getty Images)

are farmers to supply them. To encourage residents of lower-income neigh-borhoods to patronize the markets, many vendors have terminals that accept EBT. Most markets are seasonal and are open only one day a week, but they provide an important source of local foods, and an opportunity for people to mingle and socialize in ways that supermarkets do not encourage. Seasons are marked with food. Strawberries, asparagus, and peas announce the end of a long winter. In July, people chat while shucking corn. Tomatoes invite careful prodding. As New Yorkers have developed more sophisticated palates, and as Greenmarkets have ranged into more diverse neighborhoods, basil and cucumbers are now side by side with Asian greens, wasabi sprouts, cilantro and culantro, and freshly jarred kimchi. Growing concerns about factory-farmed meat have created a market for lamb, chicken, beef, and pork. Cus-tomers can talk to producers, learning why some grow organically while others bypass certification and depend on their customers' trust.

Supermarkets vary greatly by neighborhood. Whole Foods, with its full range of grass-fed beef, organic chicken, line-caught fish, and beautifully dis-played produce, cheeses, and coffees, locates in well-to-do neighborhoods with high foot traffic like Columbus Circle, Union Square, and Chelsea. Shopping at Whole Foods duplicates the experience of wandering a market, while offering prices on basic goods that are comparable to those in less-luxurious grocery stores. Trader Joe's has wide appeal for their relatively low-cost prepared foods and snacks. They, too, are found only in well-to-do neighborhoods. Fairway's original store is on the Upper West Side. They have since opened stores in Harlem and in Red Hook, Brooklyn. Here, shopping is a contact sport, with great prices on produce combined with gourmet goods and a full-service butcher and fishmonger. In these "better" neighborhoods, even the national chains like Pathmark are nicely appointed and offer a wide selection of products.

In low- and moderate-income neighborhoods, supermarkets are run-down, selling tired-looking produce and limited selections of meat and poultry. Shelves lined with processed foods reinforce the health and diet problems fac-ing residents. It is no problem finding 20 kinds of sugary cereal and juice-less fruit punch, but it is highly unlikely that these stores will carry natural peanut butter or bulk grains. The tired argument is that healthy foods will not sell in lower-income neighborhoods, but studies find over and over that residents are well aware of the dangers of unhealthy choices for their community's health. Mobility is relative; in gentrifying neighborhoods, among the signs of change are people getting off the subways carrying bags of groceries from other, more affluent parts of the city. In Washington Heights, for example, the new professional classes shop at Fairway and West Side Market; longtime residents make do with the Associated with its shabby awning, rusty carts, and constant funk of spoiled meat. The prices are higher for most goods, except for Central American and Caribbean staples like plantains.

While New York City has not joined the mayor of Rome in declaring that access to healthy food is a civil right, many changes have been made to the school lunch, and breakfast, programs. Efforts have been made to reduce the total fats, salts, and sugars in school food and to increase total nutrients and fiber. Changes are incremental. Obstacles include lack of infrastructure (schools where cafeterias are designed to reheat, not cook, food), funding, and kids' tastes. Introducing a healthy option is pointless if it ends up in the trash. Nonetheless, the Department of Education is committed to introducing more cultural variety and more locally sourced foods. All apples purchased by the school system are now grown in New York State; local carrots will soon follow. Milk is now skim, not whole or chocolate, and soy milk is available for the many children of African and Asian descent who are lactose intolerant. For many lower-income children, the meals eaten at school (free or nearly free) are the only full meals they eat. Summer programs were introduced to fill in the gaps between school terms. Ensuring that these meals are nutritionally balanced and otherwise fulfilling is critical to long-term public health and to advancing justice through access to food.

Babette Audant and Ken Albala

Further Reading

Grimes, William. *Appetite City: A Culinary History of New York*. New York: North Point Press, 2009.

Hauck-Lawson, Annie, and Jonathan Deutsch, eds. *Gastropolis: Food and New York City*. New York: Columbia University Press, 2009.

The Midwest

The American Midwest comprises 12 states: Ohio, Michigan, Indiana, Illinois, Wisconsin, Minnesota, Iowa, Missouri, Kansas, Nebraska, South Dakota, and North Dakota.

Ideas about diet and health among Midwesterners do not spring from religious tenets, with several small exceptions, but from modern science and common sense. This has not always been the case, since in the nineteenth and early twentieth centuries folk medicine and folktales were often invoked to cure illness and promote physical health. One collection of folklore from the 1930s shows that some rural people believed that goiters (a painful swelling of the thyroid gland, usually from a lack of iodine in the diet) could be cured by hanging a warty frog around the victim's neck or by boiling a frog alive and rubbing the fat on the goiter. At the same time, many herbal medicines were concocted and used locally. Sassafras tea, for instance, was widely used as a healthful tonic after a long winter when "the blood thickened" and people wanted to cleanse their systems by purging themselves. Nonetheless, in the absence of scientific research, patent medicines were also widely used, most of them sold by "quack" (phony) medical practitioners who laced their potions with lots of high-percentage alcohol.

Diet has always played an important role in people's ideas about good health. Rural people looked forward to the first wild greens of the spring and ate them as "sallets." When the first cultivated lettuces appeared, they, too, were consumed as health foods. Similar ideas about the obvious connections between diet and health drove the earliest health reformers, the most famous being Sylvester Graham in the early nineteenth century. He believed that chemical additives to foods were harmful and so promoted eating whole-grain flours. His graham cracker was widely known, though nothing like the biscuit of the same name today. His ideas were taken up by the Kellogg brothers, whose sanitarium (literally, "healthy place") in Battle Creek, Michigan, became hugely popular. People who came to restore their health ate a special diet consisting of many vegetables and high-fiber foods. One of these was corn flakes, which the Kelloggs invented and one of the brothers marketed nationally. Thus began the breakfast cereal industry, many of whose products are still marketed as important to a healthy diet. Several of the major cereal producers remain as Midwest-based companies.

If eating a good breakfast is important to health, so are other dietary procedures and products. In the present day, people in the Midwest are as concerned about diet and health as they are in other parts of the country. Overweight to the point of obesity, high blood pressure, blood serum cholesterol as a danger to the heart, and cancers are among the chief worries. As a result, and despite the notion of midwestern food being filled with saturated fats, sugars, and high amounts of gluten, people have changed their diets in the last several decades. Fat and salt consumption has decreased, and leaner meats and fruits and vegetables are eaten in greater amounts than ever. Obesity levels and other health statistics in the Midwest are about in the middle range for American states—about 26 percent of the population. Life expectancy is also at the national average. This compares favorably with statistics from 1940 when the surgeon general of Illinois issued a report stating that the average life expectancy of an average male in the state was 60 years old, without hope of it ever getting better.

The single dietary factor leading to ill health in the Midwest is poverty. The urban poor's inability to find and pay for healthy foods (high-carbohydrate, high-fat, and high-salt foods are cheaper) is matched by the lack of money for similar foods among the rural poor. Obesity rates for such people in the Midwest are among the highest in the United States, ranging up to 36 percent. Obesity leads to many other health issues, from heart attacks to respiratory problems. Individuals know this, but their circumstances do not allow for healthier diets. As such, this is a major public health problem in the United States' agricultural heartland.

Bruce Kraig

Corn Chowder

Serves 6–8

1/4 lb bacon, chopped
8 tbsp butter
2 large potatoes, diced (about 3/4 lb)
1 large carrot, sliced into rounds
1 small onion, chopped
4 ears fresh sweet corn, shucked and kernels cut from cob
Water to cover
4 tbsp flour
2 c milk
1 tsp salt, or to taste
Ground black pepper to taste

Place bacon in a deep pan over medium heat. Cook bacon until the fat melts but the bacon is not crispy. Add 4 tablespoons butter, and melt. Add potatoes, carrot, and onion, and sauté in butter and bacon until the vegetables are coated and onion begins to wilt. Add just enough water to cover, and bring to a boil. Reduce heat to a simmer, cover pan, and cook until potatoes are tender, 15–20 minutes. Meanwhile, melt 4 tablespoons butter in a separate saucepan. Whisk the flour into the butter until completely blended. Stir the milk into the butter-flour mixture until smooth.

When the vegetables are done stir them with a whisk or fork until the potatoes break up into small lumps. Stir in the milk mixture, stirring well. When thickened and heated through, add salt and pepper to taste and stir well. Serve with corn muffins or cornbread.

Further Reading

Cayton, Andrew R. L., and Susan E. Gray, eds. *The American Midwest: Essays on Regional History.* Bloomington: University of Indiana Press, 2001.

Sisson, Richard, Christian Zacher, and Andrew R. L. Cayton. *The American Midwest: An Interpretive Encyclopedia.* Bloomington: University of Indiana Press, 2007.

New England

New England comprises six states in the northeastern corner of the United States: Maine, Vermont, New Hampshire, Massachusetts, Rhode Island, and Connecticut.

Research has established that a lack of physical activity coupled with unhealthy eating patterns contributes to obesity and a number of chronic diseases, including some cancers, cardiovascular disease, and diabetes. Compared with people who consume a diet with only small amounts of fruits and vegetables, those who eat more generous amounts as part of a healthful diet are likely to have reduced risk of chronic diseases.

Americans in general have been growing heavier over the last several decades, which can be viewed in part as a trend related to living in an affluent and well-nourished society. Changes in technology have allowed a more sedentary lifestyle; in most families, both parents usually work, and the proliferation of fast food and other convenience foods, which tend to be high in fat and simple carbohydrates, has also contributed to the increasing size of the American waistline.

Compared with other Americans, New England residents are among the least obese; relatively few have a body mass index, or BMI, of greater than 30. Obesity trends upward from south to north. New Englanders struggle more with overweight—a BMI of 25–29.9. Here, the trend is reversed from north to south, with more overweight people in southern New England. The total population who are either overweight or obese is about 60 percent. Finally, about 40 percent of New Englanders are neither underweight nor overweight.

The optimal diet for maintaining good health, as established by governmental and independent studies, includes at least five servings of vegetables and fruits per day. While only about 30 percent of Americans report consuming the recommended amount, the New England states are in the top 20 of those who do so. Exercise is also a key component of good health. About 20 percent of New Englanders are considered to be at risk for health problems due to a lack of physical activity.

In recent years, medical practice in the United States is placing a greater emphasis on treating disease by prescribing lifestyle changes in diet and exercise as an adjunct to medication and other therapies. Complementary and alternative medicines are becoming more integrated into traditional medical practice. Such medicines and therapies include homeopathy and herbal medicines, mind-body balancing practices (such as yoga, meditation, or tai chi classes), acupuncture, massage and relaxation techniques, and energy healing therapies. The National Institutes of Health created the National Center for Complementary and Alternative Medicine in 1999 to advance research on such therapies and make authoritative information available to the public.

Meg Ragland

Further Reading

Carlisle, Nancy, and Melinda Talbot, with Jennifer Pustz. *America's Kitchens.* Boston: Historic New England, 2008.

McWilliams, James. *A Revolution in Eating: How the Quest for Food Shaped America.* New York: Columbia University Press, 2005.

Smith, Andrew. *Eating History: 30 Turning Points in the Making of American Cuisine.* New York: Columbia University Press, 2009.

The Pacific Northwest

The Pacific Northwest is the North American geographic region along the northeastern edge of the Pacific Ocean. It is predominantly limited to the states of Washington and Oregon in the United States and the province of British Columbia in Canada, though it often includes Idaho, western Montana, southeastern Alaska, and northern California.

The Pacific Northwestern diet is comparable to that in the rest of the United States and Canada, though it leans toward slightly healthier choices. The Pacific Northwest has a high proportion of vegetarians and vegans compared with elsewhere in the United States and Canada. Its major urban centers (Portland, Seattle, and Vancouver) are considered to be the top three vegetarian-friendly cities in North America according to surveys by the nonprofit organization People for the Ethical Treatment of Animals (PETA). Vegetarians and vegans in the Pacific Northwest tend to simply eat meatless versions of the same foods that omnivores eat or meat substitutes that are usually made of soy or textured vegetable protein (TVP). They also tend to rely more heavily on Asian cuisines, deriving much of their protein intake from tofu (soybean curd originally from China but now widespread across Asia), tempeh (fermented soy or grain cakes from Indonesia), and seitan (solid wheat gluten from China, Japan, and Vietnam). Many vegetarians add nutritional supplements to their foods as seasonings—Bragg Liquid Aminos (a salty-tasting source of 16 amino acids that resembles tamari or soy sauce) and nutritional yeast flakes (a source of B-complex vitamins that is often used for flavoring cheese substitutes) are in nearly every vegetarian kitchen in the Pacific Northwest.

Ecologically conscientious or so-called green lifestyles are common in the Pacific Northwest, and this is reflected in the dietary choices that are made by many of its residents. Organically grown produce and free-range, organic meats are readily available at most mainstream grocery stores, and specialty stores that provide a wide selection of locally grown meats and produce are relatively common, even in smaller cities. Many heirloom varieties of vegetables and fruits are grown and sold in the region, and these are more available and affordable than in other parts of the United States or Canada. Many of the region's restaurants have received accolades for taking advantage of the Pacific Northwest's bounty by showcasing local flora and fauna on their menus. Some restaurants even have their own farms.

Farmers' markets are another successful means of closing the gap between farm and table, in that the people who grow or raise the foods can sell directly to the consumer. Most neighborhoods or districts in each urban center have a farmers' market (usually open one day per week), and even smaller urban areas (especially college towns like Eugene, Oregon, and Olympia, Washington) tend to have at least one farmers' market. Community-supported agriculture, or CSAs, enable individuals or families to purchase a yearly share of a local farm's seasonal produce (sometimes delivered directly to their homes), while simultaneously providing income to small, organic farmers.

Heather Arndt-Anderson

Further Reading

Cook, Langdon. *Fat of the Land: Adventures of a 21st Century Forager.* Seattle, WA: Skipstone Press/Mountaineer Books, 2009.

Long, Lucy M. *Regional American Food Culture.* Westport, CT: Greenwood Press, 2009.

Manning, Ivy. *The Farm to Table Cookbook: The Art of Eating Locally.* Seattle, WA: Sasquatch Books, 2008

Parr, Tami. *Artisan Cheese of the Pacific Northwest: A Discovery Guide.* Woodstock, VT: Countryman Press, 2009.

The South

Five states border the Atlantic Ocean: Virginia, North Carolina, South Carolina, Georgia, and Florida; four others stretch westward from Florida, on the Gulf of Mexico: Alabama, Mississippi, Louisiana, and Texas. Two other states, Tennessee and Arkansas, connect on opposite sides of the Mississippi River and stretch westward from Virginia to Texas.

The American South has the highest rate of obesity in the United States. Despite much talk about curtailing sugar, salt, and fat, the South's middle class complicates this by dietary inconsistency, spurning low-fat seasoning meat such as smoked neck in vegetables and instead cooking bacon with brown sugar or adding sugar-laden products to a barbecue sauce. Hidden calories in condiments such as tomato sauce and prepared foods are frequently ignored, as are visible calories in starchy vegetables such as baked potatoes with sour cream.

Although the rising obesity among the poor is attributed to unhealthy home cooking—frying a pork chop, for instance, or seasoning meat in the vegetables—snacking and frequent eating in fast-food restaurants with more calories in less-filling foods are more likely the culprit. Fresh fruits and vegetables, as well as meat lower in fat, are expensive out of season. Small neighborhood grocery stores accommodating the poor tend to be more expensive or have been supplanted by stores attached to gasoline stations, which offer high-carbohydrate snacks and canned products high in salt. Food stamps have the possibility for improved nutrition and can now be used where fresh products are available, such as farmers' markets. Fad diets abound. Yet those with access to fresh food find that eating all things in moderation not only is pleasing but also, in the long run, is healthier and reduces obesity.

Nathalie Dupree

Food Processor Biscuits

2^1/$_2$ c self-rising flour
^{1}/$_2$ c shortening or lard, frozen
^{3}/$_4$–1 c milk or buttermilk

$^1/_4$–$^1/_3$ c melted butter
$^1/_4$ c all-purpose flour for shaping

Preheat the oven to 500°F. Add 2 cups of the flour to a food processor using the steel or pastry blade. Cut one-half of the shortening into $^1/_4$-inch cubes; cut the second half into $^1/_2$-inch cubes and refrigerate. Add the cold $^1/_4$-inch cubes to the food processor. Pulse one or two times until it is like cornmeal; add the remainder of the shortening and process until pea sized. Add the ¾ cup of milk. Pulse 2 or 3 times until the shortening is cut in and the milk is incorporated, looking a bit like cottage cheese. The mixture should loosely cling to a finger. Add more flour or milk as needed. Lightly flour a work surface. Pat dough to $^1/_4$ inch thick. Fold in half. Pat out again. Fold again. Repeat two more times. Pat out $^1/_4$ inch thick. Brush half the dough with the melted butter. Fold the dough over to make it 4 inches thick. Dip a 2-inch round metal cutter into the flour. Cut out rounds in the dough, starting at the outside, avoiding the fold. Move biscuits to a greased sided cookie sheet or iron skillet next to each other. Bake for 10–12 minutes on the second rack of the oven.

Further Reading

Dabney, Joseph E. *Smokehouse Ham, Spoon Bread and Scuppernong Wine*. Nashville, TN: Cumberland House, 2008.

Fowler, Damon Lee. *Classical Southern Cooking*. Salt Lake City, UT: Gibbs-Smith, 2008.

Long, Lucy M. *Regional American Food Culture*. Westport, CT: Greenwood Press, 2009.

The Southwest

The U.S. Southwest comprises the states of Arizona, Colorado, New Mexico, and Utah, including some parts of Texas.

For many Americans, Southwestern foodways are more commonly conceptualized as a cuisine marked by the heavy use of chili, fat, and meat. In modern times, health experts have watched with alarm the increased rates of obesity and type 2 diabetes among minority populations, including both Native Americans and Latinos, in the U.S. Southwest. Pointing to the traditional foodways as a culprit, public health specialists and dieticians have proposed radical changes in traditional diets, in an attempt to head off a future health disaster. Other experts call for a more judicious analysis of the food-ways of the Southwest, often citing the healthier aspects of an earlier, more traditional diet based on vegetables, complex carbohydrates, little animal fat, and no processed foods. For these food activists, drawing on the ancestral heritage of Native American, Hispanic, and Anglo frontier foodways repre-sents an opportunity to improve diets while at the same time allowing ances-tral foods to play important roles in conserving cultural heritage.

Lois Stanford

Further Reading

Abarca, Meredith. *Voices in the Kitchen: Views of Food and the World from Working-Class Mexican and Mexican American Women*. College Station: Texas A&M Press, 2006.

DeWitt, Dave. *Cuisines of the Southwest: An Illustrated Food History with More than 160 Regional Recipes*. Phoenix, AZ: Golden West, 2008.

Nabhan, Gary Paul. *Renewing America's Food Traditions: Saving and Savoring the Continent's Most Endangered Foods*. White River Junction, VT: Chelsea Green, 2008.

Venezuela

Population: 28,459,085 (July 2013 est.)
Population Rank: 45th
Population Growth Rate: 1.44% (2013 est.)
Life Expectancy at Birth: 74.23 years (2013 est.)
Health Expenditures: 5.2% of GDP (2011)
People with Access to Safe Drinking Water: 92% of population (2000 est.)
Average Daily Caloric Consumption: 2,610
Adult Obesity Rate: 30.3% (2008)
Underweight Children under Age 5: 3.7% (2007)

Early Spanish commentators noted the glowing good health of South America's indigenous peoples, including those of Venezuela. They talked of strong, healthy stature, shining hair, and gleaming teeth, properties soon to disappear with the deadly onslaught of foreign germs, slavery, and, as even sixteenth-century commentators suggested, the Spanish diet. Like all con-querors, the Spanish imported as much of their own diet as possible. In addi-tion to new vegetables, herbs, and wheat, they brought farm animals, fat, sugar, and the expectation of three meals a day. They taught the local population to fry their foods in lard.

In terms of flavors and technology, the Spanish contribution merged with indigenous ingredients and techniques and gave birth to cocina criolla, something greater than the sum of its parts. But today the cuisines of Venezuela and other Latin American countries are much higher in fat and sugar than those of the pre-Hispanic period. Frying is widely used. Sugary sodas are as popular as fruit juices. Those with enough money now confront the evils of the Western diet. At the same time, class distinctions leave some people with too little money to buy meats, fats, and sweets in any large quantity and others with too little to eat at all. Only in the last decade have Venezuelans connected the dots between overconsumption of animal fats and ill health. Within recent years, the use of lard has declined while vegetable oils have rallied, hopefully a first step in a healthier direction.

Nancy G. Freeman

Further Reading

Dineen, Mark. *Culture and Customs of Venezuela.* Westport, CT: Greenwood Press, 2001.

Lovera, José Rafael. *Food Culture in South America.* Westport, CT: Greenwood Press, 2005.

Asia and Oceania

Aboriginal Australians

The diet of the average Aboriginal Australian family has been modified drastically over the past 200 years; a brief history of this change is warranted to understand the modern Aboriginal Australian diet. Traditional Aboriginal Australian cuisine was based on the belief that people should live in harmony with their environment instead of damaging it, as well as a practice of seasonal eating. As hunter-gatherers, they would travel around based on the season and available food supply, and as a result, they often ate fresher food, which is healthier than processed food. This also helped prevent them from completely depleting a food supply in a single area, as they constantly moved to find new food sources. Through trial and error, they discovered foods that hurt their bodies and foods that increased their health, and they passed this knowledge down to younger generations through songs and stories.

The Europeans settled in the country in the late eighteenth century and took ownership of the land because they assumed it was *terra nullius,* a legal term that means "owned by no one." Aboriginal Australian clans were displaced or killed as Europeans spread out for settlements and to raise herds and grow crops. Life as hunter-gatherers taught Aboriginals to adapt to new environments, and they coped by hunting the herds and cooking them using traditional methods, as well as hunting newly introduced vermin like rabbits that were killing off native animals.

Shortly after European settlement, the newly formed government started handing out rations of Western food to displaced Aboriginal Australians, and they quickly became dependent on the handouts. Other Aboriginals were sent to work at pastoral stations where they received similar rations in exchange for work—foods they had never tried such as corned beef, flour, sugar, and tea. At this point, Aboriginal diets depended largely on how well the station stores were stocked. If the station store manager was not empathetic to the Aboriginals, the store would lack healthy, nutritious food, which negatively affected Aboriginal health, as the foods available were low in calcium and vitamins. They shifted from a mainly vegetarian diet to a meat-focused diet because rations rarely had fruit, vegetables, and dairy, due to poor transportation methods and a lack of refrigeration.

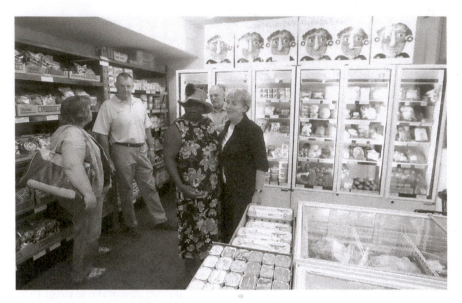

This store offers healthy, fresh food for the aboriginal population of the Northern Territory of Australia. (Glenn Campbell/The Sydney Morning Herald/ Fairfax Media/Getty Images)

Families were separated, and from the late eighteenth through the late nineteenth century, Australian federal and state governments removed Aboriginal children from their homes and placed them into European Australian households, which made it difficult to pass on the oral culture and culinary traditions of their people. However, this did not eliminate Aboriginal Australian culinary culture completely; some remote-living Aboriginals adapted by finding time to hunt and gather traditional *bush tucker* (Aboriginal food) on the weekends, and when work on the stations would slow down, many would go on a walkabout, or a spiritual walk into the bush to live off the land, rebuild their health and strength, and share Aboriginal traditions.

In the late 1960s Aboriginal civil rights were finally recognized, and government control over where they lived and moved was taken away. Many Aboriginal Australian workers were let go from their station jobs and forced to live in fringe camps and be on welfare, which only further cemented their dependence on processed foods that were cheap and easily available in local stores. There was also a decline in gathering bush tucker, which was exacerbated by the ongoing clearing of land for more settlement areas.

From the 1960s until the present, Aboriginal clans and families have taken various paths that have ultimately led them to one of two destinations: living in a rural, remote Aboriginal community, often close to the outback, or moving closer to cities and towns and attempting to assimilate even more into Western society. Those who created their own remote Aboriginal communities still rely on station stores or monthly mail trucks for their food supplies. Canned fruit, powdered milk, rice, and canned meat are staples in a modern remote Aboriginal diet. But ever-adaptive, remote-living Aboriginals have combined parts of Western culture with their traditional culture, supplementing processed foods with Aboriginal foods and cooking methods whenever possible. Many families adapt popular recipes from other ethnic cuisines to their native food supply and cooking methods, and curried *gulah*, or spaghetti and kangaroo meatballs, is commonly found in modern Aboriginal campsites. Bush plum pudding is another common recipe found in campsites during the holidays, an Aboriginal take on the popular British Christmas dish.

Those Aboriginal families who chose to live closer to Western society had better exposure to food sources in the form of grocery stores, which meant direct access to fresh fruit, vegetables, and dairy. But meat and sugar still play a significant role in their diet, just as they did at the pastoral stations. Even though Aboriginals living in a nonremote area can now self-select their diet for the first time in 100 years, they still cling to their learned pastoral station diets because that is what they know. Fast-food outlets are also finding their way into the average modern nonremote Aboriginal diet. Almost all of these communities (remote and nonremote) are lower class or impoverished, so food supplies vary based on the money a family or community can generate at any given time.

An interesting twist in the history of Aboriginal Australian cuisine is the native-foods industry of Australia. Created in the 1970s, the native-foods industry comprises indigenous Australian foods such as fruits, spices, nuts, and herbs, commercially manufactured for restaurants and gourmet stores. A positive side of the Australian native-foods industry is that it utilizes Aboriginal cultural heritage and provides Aboriginals with jobs. However, most native foods are so high priced that neither remote nor nonremote Aboriginal families can afford to work them into their regular diets.

Due to the Westernization of their diets to varying degrees, both remote-living and urban-dwelling Aboriginal Australians have a number of serious health concerns, including obesity, diabetes, cardiovascular disease, and alcohol and drug abuse. As of 2005, 57 percent of Aboriginal Australians were overweight or obese regardless of whether they lived in a city or the bush.

They are 1.2 times more likely to be overweight or obese compared with their nonindigenous counterparts.

Studies show that Aboriginal Australian babies are fully nourished by their mother's milk, but with so much processed food in their environment, they inevitably gain excess weight and become unhealthy when they move on to solid foods. Exercise is another large factor in why so many Aboriginals are overweight, as more than 70 percent of remote and nonremote Aboriginal Australians do little to no exercise. Diet and exercise are also contributors to the large number of Aboriginals suffering from cardiovascular disease and high blood pressure.

One group trying to make a difference in Aboriginal Australian health is the Fred Hollows Foundation, which has been collaborating with indigenous women in the Northern Territory to create a cookbook for indigenous Australians that can be used in remote communities and can help alleviate poor health due to diet. Aboriginal Australians' increased rate of obesity has led to an excessive occurrence of type 2 diabetes in the Aboriginal Australian community, making them four times more likely to develop diabetes than the nonindigenous Australian community. The first Aboriginal Australian case of diabetes occurred in 1923, but before that, there was no history of metabolic conditions among this community, as most hunter-gatherer Aboriginals were in good physical condition and their diet was healthy. After a group of diabetic Aboriginal Australians returned to a traditional lifestyle and cuisine, studies found that their health improved and their diabetes symptoms either lessened or disappeared. Alcohol is another factor in poor Aboriginal health, specifically in diabetes and cardiovascular disease. Studies have shown that although Aboriginals are less apt to drink alcohol than nonindigenous Australians, they are more prone to drink dangerous amounts of alcohol when they do imbibe. Between 2000 and 2004, injuries or diseases related to alcohol use led to the deaths of 1,145 Aboriginal Australians, with the median age of death around 35 years of age.

Leena Trivedi-Grenier

Further Reading

"Australia's Disturbing Health Disparities Set Aboriginals Apart." *Bulletin of the World Health Organization* 86, No. 4 (2008): 241–320.

Haden, Roger. *Food Culture in the Pacific Islands.* Westport, CT: Greenwood Press, 2009.

Ramsden, Jessica. "Australia's Native Cuisine: A Study of Food in Contemporary Australian Society." Master's thesis, University of Adelaide, 2008.

Afghanistan

Population: 31,108,077 (July 2013 est.)
Population Rank: 40th
Population Growth Rate: 2.25% (2013 est.)
Life Expectancy at Birth: 50.11 years (2013 est.)
Health Expenditures: 9.6% of GDP (2011)
People with Access to Safe Drinking Water: 50% of population (2010 est.)
Average Daily Caloric Consumption: Unknown
Adult Obesity Rate: 2.2% (2008)
Underweight Children under Age 5: 32.9% (2004)

Although much liked by Afghans, meat is expensive and sometimes eaten only once or twice a week. However, the bread is very nutritious, and when supplemented with soups, pulses, and vegetables it provides enough protein, carbohydrates, vitamins, and minerals for a fairly healthy diet. Desserts and sweets are a luxury, but fruits abound in summer and autumn. Afghan tastes favor a large amount of fat or oil in their cooking. Indeed, this is a sort of status symbol. Many Afghans, especially those now living in the West, have reduced their use of oil or fat and are much more conscious about a healthy diet.

Many people in Afghanistan still adhere in everyday life to the ancient Persian concept of *sardi/garmi,* literally "cold/hot." Like yin-yang in China, it is a system for classifying foods for the purpose of dietary health. In general people believe that eating "hot" foods can alleviate "cold" illnesses such as the common cold. "Cold" foods are prescribed to reduce fevers or hot tempers. "Hot" and "cold" here refer to the properties of the food, not the temperature. While there are some differences of opinion as to just what foods can be classified as hot or cold, there is a definite pattern. Hot foods are rich, warm in aroma, sweet, and high in calories and carbohydrates, whereas cold foods are generally characterized by acidity or blandness, have a high water content, and are low in calories. In Afghanistan hot foods include sugar and honey, fats and oils, wheat flour and chickpea flour, dried fruits, nuts, garlic and onions, fish, meat, eggs, and most spices such as chilies, fenugreek, ginger, turmeric, and saffron. Cold foods include rose water, milk and yogurt, chicken, rice, some pulses (such as lentils and kidney beans), fresh fruits (such as melons, grapes, pears, apples, and lemons) and vegetables (especially spinach, cucumbers, and lettuce), and most herbs (such as cilantro and dill). Both spices and herbs are valued by Afghans for their medicinal properties, and many are used to aid digestion or help cure and alleviate other illnesses.

Helen Saberi

Burani Bonjon

2–3 large eggplants
Vegetable oil for frying
1 medium onion, finely chopped
2 medium tomatoes, thinly sliced
1 green bell pepper, finely sliced in rings (optional)
Salt
$^1/_4$–$^1/_2$ tsp red pepper
1–2 c strained yogurt
2 cloves garlic, peeled and crushed
2 tsp dried mint

Peel the eggplants, and slice them into rounds about $^1/_4$–$^1/_2$ inch thick.

Heat plenty of vegetable oil in a frying pan (eggplant soaks up a lot of oil), and fry as many slices of the eggplant as possible in one layer. Fry on both sides until brown. Remove from the pan, and drain on absorbent kitchen paper. Repeat with the remaining eggplant, adding more oil as necessary.

Fry the chopped onions in a little oil until reddish-brown. Arrange the eggplant, sliced tomatoes, and sliced pepper in layers in the frying pan, sprinkling each layer with some fried onion and a little salt and a little red pepper. Spoon over 2–3 tablespoons of water, cover the pan with a lid, and simmer over low heat for about 20 to 30 minutes.

Meanwhile, combine the strained yogurt, the crushed garlic, a little salt, and the dried mint. Put half of the strained yogurt onto a warm serving dish. Carefully remove the eggplant from the pan with a spatula, and arrange it on the yogurt. Dot the rest of the yogurt over the eggplant, and sprinkle over any remaining sauce (but not the oil) from the eggplant on top. Serve immediately with freshly baked nan or with chalau.

Further Reading

Saberi, Helen. *Noshe Djan: Afghan Food and Cookery.* Devon, UK: Prospect Books, 2000.

Saberi, Helen. "Travel and Food in Afghanistan." In *Food on the Move, Proceedings of the Oxford Symposium on Food and Cookery, 1996,* edited by Harlan Walker. Devon, UK: Prospect Books, 1997.

Australia

Population: 22,262,501 (July 2013 est.)
Population Rank: 57th
Population Growth Rate: 1.11% (2013 est.)
Life Expectancy at Birth: 81.98 years (2013 est.)
Health Expenditures: 9% of GDP (2011)
People with Access to Safe Drinking Water: 100% of population (2010 est.)
Average Daily Caloric Consumption: 3,190
Adult Obesity Rate: 26.8% (2008)
Underweight Children under Age 5: Unknown or Negligible

At the turn of the century, 60 percent of Australians age 25 and over were overweight, and 21 percent were obese. Both adult and childhood obesity continue to be a growing concern in Australia. As in most Western countries, Australians seem to be suffering from what Australian thinker and author Clive Hamilton has diagnosed as "affluenza" and the overindulgences associated with an office-bound, consumption-based lifestyle. Whether Australians blame the influx of American fast-food chains over the last 30 years, the long heritage of a starchy, meat-filled British diet, or the abundance of homegrown meat pies and take-out fish-and-chip shops more suited to an earlier, more active era, they are looking for solutions among the varied cuisines around them. Almost since settlement, Australians have discussed the merits of following a Mediterranean diet in their largely Mediterranean climate, as a matter of health. These discussions continue today. Added to them are recognitions of the health benefits Asian and other cuisines have to offer. Australians are doing what they have always done to answer the perceived health crisis: they are looking across the world for solutions they can cook at home, casting off what does not fit and wrangling what does into patterns of cooking that work in a "she'll be right" functional, fast-moving, and avidly discussed Australian cuisine.

Andrea MacRae

Further Reading

Santich, Barbara. "The High and the Low: Australian Cuisine in the Late Nineteenth and Early Twentieth Centuries." *Journal of Australian Studies* 30, No. 87 (2006): 43.

Santich, Barbara. "Paradigm Shifts in the History of Dietary Advice in Australia." *Nutrition and Dietetics* 62, No. 4 (2005): 152–57.

Symons, Michael. *One Continuous Picnic*. 1982. Carlton, Australia: Melbourne University Press, 2007.

Bangladesh

Population: 163,654,860 (July 2013 est.)
Population Rank: 8th
Population Growth Rate: 1.59% (2013 est.)
Life Expectancy at Birth: 70.36 years (2013 est.)
Health Expenditures: 3.7% of GDP (2011)
People with Access to Safe Drinking Water: 81% of population (2010 est.)
Average Daily Caloric Consumption: 2,250
Adult Obesity Rate: 1.1% (2008)
Underweight Children under Age 5: 41.3% (2007)

In addition to Western medicine, the traditional Ayurvedic and Unani systems are widely practiced in Bangladesh, especially at the primary health care level. An estimated 70 to 75 percent of people in the country still use traditional medicine to manage their health problems.

Ayurveda, the ancient Indian school of medicine, had its roots in the region. Ayurveda is holistic: it treats the entire individual, including one's mental, emotional, and physical makeup, not just the symptoms. Ayurveda also strongly emphasizes the link between health and diet. The goal of eating is to increase desirable qualities, reduce negative qualities, and introduce previously absent qualities.

Unani, the Muslim system of medicine, is offered by 4,000 qualified and professionally trained physicians, called *hakims*. Unani medicine is based on the humoral theory of Greek medicine, which assumes the presence of four humors in the body: blood, phlegm, yellow bile, and black bile. Every person is born with a unique humoral constitution, which represents his or her healthy state and determines his or her personality. When the amounts of the humors are changed and thrown out of balance with each other, it leads to disease. Restoring the quality and balance of humors is the goal of treatment, and diet plays a role in this. Certain foods are prescribed for certain ailments.

Colleen Taylor Sen

Further Reading

Banerji, Chitrita. *Life and Food in Bengal.* Delhi: Penguin Books India, 1991.

Sen, Colleen Taylor, with Joe Roberts. "A Carp Wearing Lipstick: The Role of Fish in Bengali Cuisine and Culture." In *Fish: Food from the Waters, Proceedings of the Oxford Symposium on Food and Cookery,* edited by Harlan Walker. Totnes, Devon, UK: Prospect Books, 1997.

Brunei

Population: 415,717 (July 2013 est.)

Population Rank: 174th

Population Growth Rate: 1.67% (2013 est.)

Life Expectancy at Birth: 76.57 years (2013 est.)

Health Expenditures: 2.5% of GDP (2011)

People with Access to Safe Drinking Water: Unknown

Average Daily Caloric Consumption: 2,990

Adult Obesity Rate: 7.5% (2008)

Underweight Children under Age 5: Unknown or Negligible

The spices and herbs used in Brunei, Malaysia, and Indonesia have been used for centuries for their health-giving properties, long before people started using them in cooking. Spices like turmeric, cinnamon, ginger juice, the Asian pennywort or *gotu kola,* and asafetida are now being seriously researched to determine their healing properties as the locals have used them for centuries with positive results. Brunei is also a well-informed country, where health authorities remind the people of health issues, such as the dangers of the cholesterol in coconut milk, and encourage active exercise classes. In BSB, the capital city, many gymnasiums offer affordable exercise classes to encourage the younger office workers to keep trim. Brunei has its fair share of joggers and Hash House Harriers, as in any part of the world, but unless the sedentary lifestyle gets to them, balanced meals with large helpings of vegetables will continue to be advantageous to health.

Carol Selva Rajah

Further Reading

Selva Rajah, Carol. *The Essential Guide to Buying and Using Essential Asian Ingredients.* Chatswood, Australia: New Holland Press, 2002.

Selva Rajah, Carol. *Heavenly Fragrance: Mastering the Art of Aromatic Asian Cooking.* Singapore: Periplus, 2008.

Cambodia

Population: 15,205,539 (July 2013 est.)
Population Rank: 68th
Population Growth Rate: 1.67% (2013 est.)
Life Expectancy at Birth: 63.41 years (2013 est.)
Health Expenditures: 5.7% of GDP (2011)
People with Access to Safe Drinking Water: 64% of population (2010 est.)
Average Daily Caloric Consumption: 2,250
Adult Obesity Rate: 2.1% (2008)
Underweight Children under Age 5: 29% (2011)

There are few food cultures more ideally suited to human health than the Cambodian diet based on rice, fish, fresh vegetables, and fruit. However, the war years disrupted the development of the once-famous Cambodian cuisine associated with the ancient Khmer Empire.

Cambodia faces severe problems with malnutrition, with many communities and households eating less than the minimal calories recommended. Most of the available calories come from rice. The World Food Program estimates that a third of the population is undernourished. The infant mortality rate of 98 deaths per 1,000 live births is dropping, as is the under-five mortality rate (143 per 1,000). But malnutrition remains a significant problem in the country. International assistance has focused on immunizations, food supplements in schools, and vitamin A supplementation. Few households use iodized salt, which means that iodine deficiency and goiter are still common.

When Cambodians fled their country as refugees, escaping war and the repressive regime of the Khmer Rouge, healers known as Khru Khmer offered a variety of traditional medical services in the refugee camps, including massage and herbal therapies.

Penny Van Esterik

Caramelized Fish

This technique of caramelizing fish is also popular in Vietnamese cooking; the caramelizing process probably has its origin in French techniques.

1 trout, cleaned and filleted
3 tbsp sugar
1 tbsp water plus 1 c water

2 cloves garlic, chopped
1 tbsp fish sauce
Black pepper
3 green onions, chopped

Cut fish into strips and set aside. Make a caramel sauce by browning 1 tablespoon sugar in 1 tablespoon water in a skillet. When it is brown, slowly add 1 cup water and stir until it is an even brown color. Add chopped garlic, the remaining sugar, and fish sauce, along with the fish steaks. Simmer, and turn the fish when it is cooked on one side and the sauce thickens. Remove from heat, and garnish with black pepper and green onions. Serve with rice.

Further Reading

Alford, Jeffrey, and Naomi Duguid. *Hot Sour Salty Sweet.* Toronto, Canada: Random House Canada, 2000.

Van Esterik, Penny. *Food Culture in Southeast Asia.* Westport, CT: Greenwood Press, 2008.

Central Asia

Kyrgyzstan

Population: 5,548,042 (July 2013 est.)
Population Rank: 112th
Population Growth Rate: 0.97% (2013 est.)
Life Expectancy at Birth: 69.75 years (2013 est.)
Health Expenditures: 6.2% of GDP (2010)
People with Access to Safe Drinking Water: 90% of population (2010 est.)
Average Daily Caloric Consumption: 2,670
Adult Obesity Rate: 15.5% (2008)
Underweight Children under Age 5: 2.7% (2006)

Tajikistan

Population: 7,910,041 (July 2013 est.)
Population Rank: 96th
Population Growth Rate: 1.79% (2013 est.)

Life Expectancy at Birth: 66.72 years (2013 est.)
Health Expenditures: 5.8% of GDP (2011)
People with Access to Safe Drinking Water: 64% of population (2010 est.)
Average Daily Caloric Consumption: 2,130
Adult Obesity Rate: 8.6% (2008)
Underweight Children under Age 5: 15% (2005)

Turkmenistan

Population: 5,113,040 (July 2013 est.)
Population Rank: 118th
Population Growth Rate: 1.15% (2013 est.)
Life Expectancy at Birth: 69.16 years (2013 est.)
Health Expenditures: 2.7% of GDP (2011)
People with Access to Safe Drinking Water: 83% of population (2000 est.)
Average Daily Caloric Consumption: 2,750
Adult Obesity Rate: 13.2% (2008)
Underweight Children under Age 5: Unknown or negligible

Uzbekistan

Population: 28,661,637 (July 2013 est.)
Population Rank: 44th
Population Growth Rate: 0.94% (2013 est.)
Life Expectancy at Birth: 73.03 years (2013 est.)
Health Expenditures: 5.4% of GDP (2011)
People with Access to Safe Drinking Water: 87% of population (2010 est.)
Average Daily Caloric Consumption: 2,530
Adult Obesity Rate: 15.1% (2008)
Underweight Children under Age 5: 4.4% (2006)

Central Asia, including the province of Xinjiang in China, is a massive territory, more than half the size of the United States. The newly independent states of Uzbekistan, Turkmenistan, Tajikistan, and Kyrgyzstan are situated east of the Caspian Sea, west of China, south of Russia, and north of Afghanistan and Iran.

In Central Asia, food is not only treated as a source of nourishment and fuel but also valued for its preventative and curative role. Specific nutritional problems include the lack of affordability of certain healthful and essential food items, the suspect quality of some foodstuffs, and the absence of public awareness of what constitutes a healthful and balanced diet.

Vitamin A and C deficiencies are common in Kyrgyzstan because the people eat fewer fruits and vegetables than do Uzbeks, Tajiks, and Turkmen. One concern in Tajikistan is the prevalence of thyroid deficiencies due to a lack of iron in the diet. Turkmen depend heavily on bread for calories, with only seasonal consumption of vegetables and fruit, resulting in a deficiency of protein and fat. Overall per capita food consumption in Uzbekistan actually increased between 1992 and 1996, except for milk products. Uzbek consumption of meat increased, while bread intake has remained relatively stable since 1992.

Central Asians loosely maintained a diet based on the ancient Greek humoral practices as propagated by the Muslim philosopher ibn Sina (born near Bukhara in Uzbekistan) in the eleventh century. This theory holds that the body has four humors (blood, yellow bile, black bile, and phlegm) that determine health and disease. The humors were, in turn, associated with the four elements: air, fire, earth, and water, which were neatly paired with the qualities hot, cold, dry, and moist. According to that theory, a proper and evenly balanced combination of humors characterized the health of the body and mind; an imbalance resulted in disease. Combining local wisdom with traditional Chinese thought, Central Asians consider foods to have either "hot" or "cold" as well as "dry" or "moist" qualities in regard to both medicinal and nutritive functions. The inextricable relationship between diet and health forms the basis for the humoral theory of medicine, which still holds considerable sway in individual food choices in the region. The layperson in Central Asia can still classify most foodstuffs as having hot or cold properties.

The major health-related problems in Central Asia are low life expectancy, cardiovascular disease, high rates of tobacco and alcohol use, and general nutritional deficiencies. These, combined with diets high in fat and low in antioxidants, mean that the conditions for cardiovascular disease are ripe. Central Asians consume well below the recommended average daily calories for the European region. Acute malnutrition among children remains high, resulting in disorders caused by lack of micronutrients such as iron and iodine. Carbohydrates in the form of bread and potatoes make up a larger part of the diet than in the past as the consumption of fats, milk products, fish, and eggs has declined. Still, the saturated fatty acids of animal fat make up a large portion of total calorie intake. According to recent reports by the World Health Organization, the Central Asian republics, while still in need of improvement, experienced some positive health results since the early

1990s. The Kyrgyz appear to have the best relative health in the region. In general, they eat a more healthful diet, smoke less, and are less frequent drinkers. Muslims in Central Asia, according to recent research, were significantly less likely to drink frequently or smoke.

Glenn R. Mack

Further Reading

Mack, Glenn R., and Asele Surina. *Food Culture of Russia and Central Asia.* Westport, CT: Greenwood Press, 2005.

Soucek, Svatopluk. *A History of Inner Asia.* Cambridge: Cambridge University Press, 2000.

China

Population: 1,349,585,838 (July 2013 est.)
Population Rank: 1st
Population Growth Rate: 0.46% (2013 est.)
Life Expectancy at Birth: 74.99 years (2013 est.)
Health Expenditures: 5.2% of GDP (2011)
People with Access to Safe Drinking Water: 91% of population (2010 est.)
Average Daily Caloric Consumption: 2,970
Adult Obesity Rate: 5.7% (2008)
Underweight Children under Age 5: 3.4% (2010)

The traditional Chinese diet of roughly milled or whole grains, vegetables, and bean curd was extremely healthy. Diabetes, heart disease, and other conditions that can be caused or made worse by food were almost unknown. A major study found that traditional Chinese almost never had these conditions, or even high blood pressure or high blood cholesterol. The only problem with the diet was getting enough to eat, but that was a major one before modern agriculture, transportation, and storage. Probably most deaths in China before 1970 were due to malnutrition or starvation, or were caused by parasites and diseases carried by polluted water and sometimes by foods themselves. Locally, some cancers were caused or made worse by poorly preserved or poorly cooked foods, or by local minerals that got into food.

Chinese medicine has always focused on food, for the very good reason that malnutrition and starvation were the commonest killers throughout most of China's history. The first recourse in illness is eating the diet considered

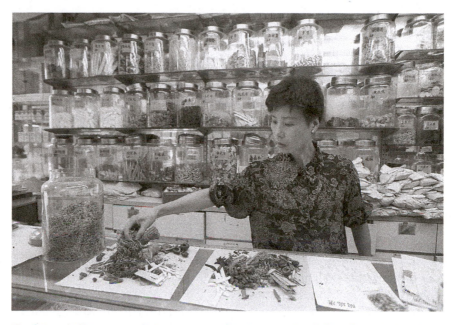

Traditional Chinese medicine purported to increase body functions during the winter. (AP Photo/Vincent Yu)

appropriate. Given this reality, it is not surprising that Chinese nutritional science reached a high level at quite early times. Medical texts more than 2,000 years old preserve nutritional lore, though of rather varying quality. Early medical books record successful nutritional therapies for beriberi (vitamin B_1 deficiency), acute diarrhea, and general debility, as well as pointing out that pine nuts are notably more conducive to long life than a primarily grain diet. (The pine nuts are high in protein and minerals lacking in grains.) The books advise a balance between yang (the hot, dry, sunny aspect of nature, dominant in males) and yin (the cool, moist, shady aspect, dominant in females). Flavors, staple grains, and other medical influences were classified in fives, the five flavors being sweet, sour, salt, bitter, and rank (possibly an early anticipation of the discovery of the umami flavor in modern times).

Basic to Chinese medicine is the concept of *qi* (pronounced "chee"), literally "air" or "breath" but expanded to include the vital spirits thought to animate and nourish the body. A good flow of qi is necessary to health. Deficiency or blockage causes disease or makes it worse. So does imbalance between yang and yin (types of qi) or between any other forms of qi. Much (perhaps, theoretically, all) Chinese medical treatment involves getting the qi back in order, as well as more direct symptomatic treatment.

The Greek school of medicine that traces back to Hippocrates (fifth century BCE) and was perfected by Galen (ca. 129–210 CE) reached China fairly early from the Near East and fused with Chinese concepts; the fusion process appears in sixth- and seventh-century medical texts. Galen's concern with hot, cool, dry, and wet naturally fused with the yang-yin concept and complemented the fivefold classification system.

Foods continued to be classified in all these ways, climaxing in the great herbal *Bencao Gangmu* by Li Shizhen (ca. 1593 CE). However, ordinary people found the heating-cooling, yang-yin dimension much more salient and useful than the others. Today, traditional Chinese still think in these terms. Heating foods are, most obviously, those that provide the most calories (literal heat energy for the body). These are fatty foods, very sweet foods, baked foods, strong alcohol, and the like. One can also understand why foods that cause burning sensations, like chili, black pepper, and ginger, are "heating." Also cataloged among the hot foods are those with "hot" colors: red beans or brown sugar. Cooling foods are those that are very low in calories (like most vegetables), those that feel "cooling" in the sense of being astringent and puckery, and those that are very watery—getting wet chills you, and drinking cold water cools you down, so watery foods are thought to be cooling. Also cooling are things that are cold colors (green or icy white, for example), especially if they look like ice (for example, rock sugar, white radishes). The perfect balance point is cooked rice, and anything similar to it—white potatoes, white-fleshed fish, soup noodles— is also considered to be at the balanced or temperate point.

The more heating foods tend to be served in winter, when people need the calories, and also at feasts, which are "hot" occasions (consider the English phrase "a hot time"). The more cooling foods go best in summer. This is especially true of foods like watermelon and cucumber that are genuinely cooling. They stay cool during the day and in prerefrigeration times were about the only things that did in China's blistering summers.

On the whole, this system kept people healthy. The classic "hot" condition was scurvy, which seems like burning. It involves redness, rash, sores, infections, constipation, and other things that seem like the result of too much heat. It was cured by eating cooling foods, notably vegetables. It is actually caused by a lack of vitamin C, which abounds in Chinese vegetables, so these foods really did cure it. Conversely, the commonest "cold" conditions were anemia (iron deficiency) and tuberculosis; they involve pallor, weakness, and often a low body temperature. Anemia is cured, and tuberculosis can be alleviated, by eating strengthening foods seen as "warming," notably red meat and organ meats. Empirically, the Chinese found that things like pig liver and wild duck meat—particularly rich sources of iron—were especially effective. Some attention was paid to drying and wetting foods, but they remained minor in the system.

Far more important was the purely Chinese concept, over 2,000 years old and probably much older, of *bupin*, "supplementing foods." These are foods that are high in protein and minerals but low in fats and carbohydrates, and thus easy to digest while extremely nourishing. They are particularly recommended for women who have just given birth, for anyone convalescing from major injury or sickness, and for elders who want to stay as hale as possible. They were originally things like pork, pig liver, duck, and game meats generally. At some point Chinese doctors found that certain odd items like tendons, mushrooms, sea cucumbers, and similar sea life worked well, and they generalized to assume that anything similar to these was a bupin. Moreover, it was logical to suppose that the odder an item looked, the more it might help, because there was a belief that odd appearance showed an abundance of qi. Thus, odd-seeming items like edible bird's nests (the nests of a tropical swift that secretes a proteinaceous substance), ancient misshapen fungi, and weird-looking or rare animals (turtles, raccoons, or dogs, for example) are considered bupin. In recent years this has proved a disaster for the species in question. Traditional conservation and management measures, very effective in many cases, have been abandoned, and overhunting is wiping out everything even remotely bupin. Perhaps the biggest irony is that none of these oddities works any better than—or, indeed, as well as—the traditional red meat and pork liver. People rarely eat bupin unless they feel the need, and modern medicine is replacing the more exotic ones.

The bupin belief grades into a belief in the magical power of some powerful animals like tigers and stags. Air-breathing catfish, which can live out of water and are very difficult to kill, are cooked as a cancer remedy, in hopes that they will transfer their tenacity of life to the patient. Another important belief is the idea that some foods are cleansing (*jing*). These are largely herbal remedies that, when taken in medicinal tea, make the body feel refreshed, cooled, and harmonized. So far, very little research has investigated their actual effects on the system. They do not "clean one out" in the sense of purgatives and emetics—both well known to the Chinese and considered a wholly separate matter.

An example of successful nutritional therapy that is being discovered worldwide is the Chinese wolfthorn plant, *gouqi* in Chinese (*Lycium chinense*). This common shrub has edible but tasteless leaves and small berries that are similar to and closely related to small tomatoes. The leaves and berries have the distinction of being among the richest in vitamins and minerals of any common food. They are thus grown for tonic use, typically in stews of pork, pork liver, Chinese wine, ginger, black vinegar, and other nutritious and strengthening items. These stews are fed to women who have just given birth and to convalescents. A significant percentage of Chinese living today owe their lives to them. The berries, dried, were always a staple of Chinese medicine stores. Recently they have appeared in markets worldwide. From the United States to Australia, one can now buy a pound bag of goji berries at the corner store, at least if the corner store has much selection of dried fruit. Another nutraceutical that has gone worldwide is wormwood (*Artemisia* spp.). It is used in China to kill intestinal worms and other parasites, including the organisms that cause malaria. One active ingredient, artemisinin, is now the drug of choice for malaria in much of the world.

E. N. Anderson

Further Reading

Campbell, T. Colin, with Thomas M. Campbell II. *The China Study.* Dallas, TX: Benbella Books, 2005.

Cheung, Sidney, and Tan Chee-Beng. *Food and Foodways in Asia: Resource, Tradition and Cooking.* London: Routledge, 2007.

Hu Shiu-ying. *Food Plants of China.* Hong Kong: Chinese University of Hong Kong, 2005.

Newman, Jacqueline. *Food Culture in China.* Westport, CT: Greenwood Press, 2004.

Hmong

Food and diet, health and disease, are controversial topics within the Hmong refugee community. Some of the older people try to maintain a traditional diet, but so much has changed that it seems impossible. For example, pork, once reserved for special occasions, is abundant, but it does not taste the same. Refrigeration, so much a part of American life, changes the flavors of food. The need to go out and work for wages results in very different time issues than when living in a village and supporting oneself by raising one's own food.

In some ways, traditional Hmong food customs, such as the emphasis on freshness and plenty of vegetables, help keep the group healthy. But others, such as a perceived value in being fat (a sign of plenty) and the uncritical acceptance of other foods, have the opposite effect. The Hmong in the United States are suffering from diseases that they did not know existed 30 years ago, and not everyone agrees on the reasons.

One of the more positive traditional practices is the tender custom of caring for a woman during the first month after the delivery of a baby. During this time, the mother is considered vulnerable and must eat a special diet for protection and to regain her strength. The diet is made up of boiled chicken with special, healing herbs. She is not allowed to work during that month, and rest is required. It is best for the husband's mother to cook and care for her daughter-in-law for the first month after delivery, which is a nice benefit for young women who, otherwise, must serve their mothers-in-law. The women say that the diet is monotonous but important. A public health study conducted by the National Institutes of Health (NIH) showed that maternal and child deaths among Hmong refugees were surprisingly low.

One negative result of the access to an abundance of food in the United States is a high rate of obesity and diabetes. In Laos, food was sometimes in short supply. There was never a surplus of food, and people adjusted to living on a low-calorie, low-fat, plant-based diet. In that environment, a fat baby was a healthy baby. When the Hmong moved to the United States, they delighted in how easy it was to have fat babies and fat children. Some of the adults also became overweight, and a high rate of diabetes, previously unknown, is the outcome. Diabetes educators find that it is difficult to work with Hmong patients, because their cultural beliefs are in conflict with Western medicine. A study in Minnesota found that Hmong refugees with diabetes do not accept that it is caused by food. Rather, they see it as a result of their refugee experience, of the loss that they have suffered. In their belief system, they are "out of balance here."

Hmong American children have learned about hot dogs, hamburgers, tacos, pizza, and other Western-style foods through their school lunch programs, and they often demand those foods at home, resulting in an especially high intake of foods that are high in calories and low in nutrients. The best efforts of nutrition educators sometimes are stymied by cultural differences. For example, one public health office took care to hire a registered dietitian with a master's degree, who was Hmong and from the local community, in an earnest effort to improve the diet and health status in the area. It looked like a win-win situation, with a culturally appropriate yet scientifically trained care provider. The dietitian did her best, concentrating on prenatal health, diabetes, weight control, and heart disease, but her advice fell on deaf ears among her clientele. The reason: she came from a low-ranking clan.

There is a high level of mistrust toward American doctors. Western medicine is cold and intrusive in comparison with the more familiar shaman. Even individuals who have converted to Christianity tend to fear and avoid American doctors. To make things more difficult, there are only 13 last names, one for each clan. There is a limited number of first names as well, resulting in many people having the same name. This causes confusion at pharmacies and health clinics, resulting in treatments and prescriptions being confused on a semiregular basis. In one example, a man with kidney problems went to see his doctor. The doctor gave him an appropriate prescription, but the pharmacist got his prescription switched with that of another man with the same name. As a result, the man suffered kidney failure. His doctor suggested dialysis, but there was a rumor circulating among the Hmong that dialysis was just a way for the doctors to collect blood that they wanted to drink. The myth of the vampire doctor started during the Vietnam War and has never really gone away. The man refused treatment until he was so weak that his American friends just picked him up and carried him to the emergency room. When his wife was notified, she came to the hospital and screamed at their American friends that the doctors just wanted to kill her husband, until a nurse, who also happened to be Hmong, managed to calm her down. In this case, the man recovered, but every time a Hmong person dies in the hospital it helps perpetuate the myth of the vampire doctor.

There is a higher rate of kidney stones and kidney failure in the Hmong population than in the general population. The reasons are unclear, but one possible cause is high protein intake combined with low water intake. It is also possible that there is a genetic enzymatic imbalance that is widespread in this small population, similar to the tendency, in some families, to develop gout due to a genetic predisposition to build up uric acid in the system. Even so, the problem might be alleviated by eating less protein and drinking more water.

Most Hmong people who now live in the United States have adjusted the traditional diet to Western standards. For example, they will keep frozen meat in the home freezer, although they still prefer meats and fish that are as fresh as possible. The preference for fresh fruits and vegetables remains, however, and those foods are to be found at Hmong-owned booths at local farmers' markets, as well as from Hmong people who have moved to rural areas where they can farm. However, most Hmong homemakers still cook rice with every meal and prefer the flavor of pork to beef, seasoned with traditional spices such as coriander, lemongrass, and monosodium glutamate.

Deborah Duchon

Further Reading

Culhane-Pera, Kathleen A., Cheng Her, and Bee Her. " 'We Are Out of Balance Here': A Hmong Cultural Model of Diabetes." *Journal of Immigrant and Minority Health* 9, No. 3 (2007): 179–90.

Culhane-Pera, Kathleen A., and Mayseng Lee. " 'Die Another Day': A Qualitative Analysis of Hmong Experiences with Kidney Stones."*Hmong Studies Journal* 7 (2006): 1–34.

Yang, Kou. "An Assessment of the Hmong American New Year and Its Implications for Hmong-American Culture." *Hmong Studies Journal* 8 (2007): 1–32.

Hong Kong

Population: 7,182,724 (July 2013 est.)
Population Rank: 99th
Population Growth Rate: 0.39% (2013 est.)
Life Expectancy at Birth: 82.2 years (2013 est.)
Health Expenditures: Unknown
People with Access to Safe Drinking Water: Unknown
Average Daily Caloric Consumption: Unknown
Adult Obesity Rate: Unknown
Underweight Children under Age 5: Unknown or Negligible

To Hong Kongers, food is never eaten just for the sake of filling the belly. Every food is believed to possess innate qualities that can ultimately affect the natural balance of a body's system. When poor diet, stress, and other hazards of twenty-first-century life throw the body out of balance, Hong Kongers rely on food as medicine to put them back on track. This understanding is grounded in the Taoist principle of yin-yang. There is no positive without a negative, no light without dark, no male without female. This is true of everything in nature, including food, and only when all elements are present in equal amounts can balance and harmony be achieved. Thus, every food is ascribed a property—hot or cold, damp or dry, nourishing or neutral—and when eaten will have a corresponding effect on the body.

The structure of the basic Chinese meal is based on this idea, and ingredients are combined in recipes according to their properties. For example, bok choy on its own is very cooling and not suitable for someone with a cold or weak constitution. Cooking bok choy with ginger, which is a warming food, counterbalances this property. This is most evident in Cantonese soup recipes where complex combinations of ingredients are simmered slowly together to create tonics that are curative or prophylactic, as the case may be. Ingredients may be purchased in markets and at special herbalist shops where Chinese doctors are available to listen to patients' pulses and prescribe brews tailored to individual needs. The shops are distinguishable by the cases of dried food items that line the walls and entrances, as well as by their unique smell—briny and musty, with an undertone of bitter medicine.

Hong Kong being a busy town, there is a fast-food option for those too busy to eat right and make their own soups—herbal tea shops. They are recognizable by large copper-colored urns with taps dispensing a variety of brews. The urns are usually placed near the front of the shop, with bowls of tea already poured and available to passersby for a quick fix. If one chooses to enter and sit, a larger menu of soups and teas is available to treat everything from fatigue to poor digestion, and others claim beauty benefits. A subtype of these shops sells the popular—and expensive—turtle pudding. Made from turtle shell and a mixture of Chinese herbs, this black, mild-tasting pudding is believed to flush toxins from the body.

Karen Lau Taylor

Mock Shark's-Fin Soup

Serves 4
This popular street snack is also easy and inexpensive to make at home. All ingredients can be found in well-stocked Asian groceries. Be careful not to overcook the vermicelli or overthicken the soup; it will become gummy.

6 oz lean pork butt, trimmed
8 c chicken stock
2 tbsp ginger, julienned
1/2 oz dried snow ear fungus, rehydrated and shredded
6–8 shiitake mushrooms, fresh or dried and rehydrated, julienned
7 tbsp water chestnut starch
8 tbsp cold water
2 tbsp oyster sauce
2 tbsp dark soy sauce
Sesame oil and white pepper, to taste
2 packages dried vermicelli, rehydrated in cold water and cut into about 2-in. sections
2 eggs, beaten
Red rice vinegar and extra julienned ginger, to serve

Rinse and dry the pork. Blanch pork in boiling water for 5 minutes. Rinse, drain, and place in pot with chicken stock and simmer for half an hour, skimming off any foam that rises to the surface.

Remove pork from stock. Reserve stock, and set pork aside to cool, and then pull the meat apart with a fork.

Heat a little oil in a wok, and sauté ginger, snow ear fungus, and mushrooms until soft and fragrant. Add reserved stock, and bring to a boil.

Meanwhile, dissolve water chestnut starch in the water and set aside.

To the wok, add oyster sauce, soy sauce, sesame oil, and white pepper, to taste. Thicken the soup with water chestnut solution to desired consistency. Stir in vermicelli. Bring to a boil, and pour in beaten eggs, stirring quickly to create thin strands of cooked egg.

Serve hot with red rice vinegar, ginger, salt, and white pepper on the side.

Further Reading

Cheung, Sidney C. H., and Chee Beng Tan. *Food and Foodways in Asia: Resource, Tradition and Cooking.* London: Routledge, 2007.

Halvorsen, Francine. *The Food and Cooking of China: An Exploration of Chinese Cuisine in the Provinces and Cities of China, Hong Kong, and Taiwan.* New York: Wiley, 1996.

India

Population: 1,220,800,359 (July 2013 est.)
Population Rank: 2nd
Population Growth Rate: 1.28% (2013 est.)
Life Expectancy at Birth: 67.48 years (2013 est.)
Health Expenditures: 3.9% of GDP (2011)
People with Access to Safe Drinking Water: 92% of population (2010 est.)
Average Daily Caloric Consumption: 2,300
Adult Obesity Rate: 1.9% (2008)
Underweight Children under Age 5: 43.5% (2006)

"You are what you eat" is a central tenet of Indian medical and philosophical systems. The best known of these is Ayurveda (which means "science of life" in Sanskrit), the ancient indigenous Indian system of medicine that is enjoying a vogue in the West. In Ayurvedic theory, all existence is made up

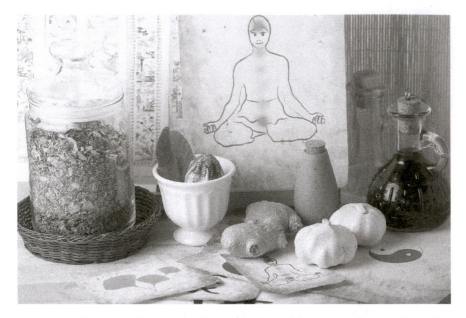

A variety of Indian herbs commonly used in the traditional healing practice of Ayurveda. (Shutterstock)

of five elements: earth, water, fire, air, and ether (or space). They in turn manifest themselves in three *doshas* that govern all human biological, psychological, and physiological functions. The doshas determine personality and disposition as well as basic constitutions. But they keep the body and mind healthy only as long as they can maintain their flow and balance. When the doshas are underproduced or overproduced, disease can result.

An important method of controlling doshas is proper eating. According to the legendary physician Charaka (b. 300 BCE), "Without proper diet, medicines are of no use; with a proper diet, medicines are unnecessary." After evaluating their patients' conditions, Ayurvedic physicians prescribe certain foods to restore the flow and balance.

Moreover, food should be "alive" in order to give life to the eater. Raw food is more alive than cooked food. Leftovers should be heated up as soon as possible or, ideally, avoided altogether. Spices should be ground freshly for each use. Ayurveda is not vegetarian; in fact, meat, especially venison, is even recommended for certain ailments, as is wine.

Once a disease has developed, it is treated by an appropriate diet recommended by the physician. This regimen always begins with fasting, "the first and most important of all medicines." Once the acute stage of the disease has passed, the patient is given appropriate medicines derived from plants and herbs. Some of these ancient remedies were later adapted by Greek and Western medicine, such as reserpine, extracted from *Wauwolfia serpentina,* which is still prescribed for reducing blood pressure.

A parallel, although distinct, attitude to food is found in yoga, which is not just a series of physical postures but a profound philosophy of life aimed at the development of a balance between body and mind in order to reunite the individual self with the Absolute. People who aspire to spiritual advancement are supposed to eat vegetarian *sattvic* foods that render the mind pure and calm—fresh fruits and vegetables, wheat, rice, cow milk, cucumber, green vegetables, nuts, and clarified butter—and avoid onion and garlic as well as meat. *Rajasic* foods, recommended for warriors, stimulate energy and creativity but also passion and aggressiveness. They include fish, chilies, wild game, goat, eggs, coffee and tea, white sugar, and spices. *Tamasic* foods fill the mind with anger, darkness, confusion, and inertia and are to be avoided. They include meat, leftovers, fast foods, fried foods and processed foods, tobacco, alcohol, and drugs.

In yet another classification that is more a part of folk medicine, all foods are classified as either "hot" or "cold" and are to be eaten or avoided depending on the time of year, an individual's constitution and state of health, and other factors. However, there is no consistency or logic in the way foods are classified as hot or cold, and there are wide regional variations. For example, most lentils are considered cold foods in western India but hot foods in the north.

Muslims practice their own system of medicine, called Unani, which is based on the humoral theory of Greek medicine that assumes the presence of four humors in the body that determine physical health and temperament. Digestion plays a central role, and minor and even some major ailments can be prevented by eating certain foods and eating in a proper manner. People are also advised to eat foods that have the opposite quality to their temperament.

Colleen Taylor Sen

Further Reading

Bharadwaj, Monisha. *The Indian Pantry.* London: Kyle Cathie, 1995.

Burnett, David, and Helen Saberi. *The Road to Vindaloo: Curry Books and Curry Cooks.* Totnes, UK: Prospect Books, 2008.

Sen, Colleen Taylor. *Food Culture in India.* Westport, CT: Greenwood Press, 2004.

Indonesia

Population: 251,160,124 (July 2013 est.)
Population Rank: 4th
Population Growth Rate: 0.99% (2013 est.)
Life Expectancy at Birth: 71.9 years (2013 est.)
Health Expenditures: 2.7% of GDP (2011)
People with Access to Safe Drinking Water: 82% of population (2010 est.)
Average Daily Caloric Consumption: 2,540
Adult Obesity Rate: 4.8% (2008)
Underweight Children under Age 5: 19.6% (2007)

While there are approximately 2.56 physicians per 1,000 people in the United States, the physician-patient ratio is much lower in Indonesia, only 0.13 physicians per 1,000 people, according to 2006 statistics. People, especially rural women in Indonesia, primarily rely on home remedies to prevent and treat illness within the family. *Dukun* (traditional healers) also play an important role in the traditional medicine system.

Jamu is a traditional herbal medicine commonly consumed by Indonesians. Different types of jamu are used to maintain physical fitness, as well as to cure certain kinds of illness. Jamu has been sold in the form of powders, creams, pills, and capsules, and its market has expanded to outside of the country. The ingredients include ginger, cinnamon, turmeric, galangal, papaya leaf, and guava leaves and flowers.

Research has shown that some pregnant women consume *jamu cabe puyang,* which reduces tiredness; bitter jamu (*jamu pahitan*), which increases appetite; and *jamu sawanan,* which prevents disease. However, some women avoid the use of jamu during pregnancy to avoid possible side effects, including the contamination of the amniotic fluid.

Similar to other developing countries, Indonesia is experiencing a nutrition transition, which is characterized by rapid changes in dietary habits, as well as a double burden of disease, in which noncommunicable diseases are becoming more prevalent while infectious diseases remain undefeated. Indonesia's leading causes of death have shifted from infectious diseases to more chronic diseases, especially cardiovascular disease. In 2002, cardiovascular disease was the leading cause of death, accounting for 22 percent of all mortality. Infectious diseases such as tuberculosis and lower respiratory infections remain major causes of death in Indonesia. Diarrheal diseases and pneumonia are still leading causes of death among children under five. In general, there has been a rapid increase in consumption of meat, eggs, milk, and processed foods, while the consumption of cereal products has decreased.

There has also been a nutrition transition for indigenous people, who used to be foragers. For example, the Punan people who reside in Kalimantan have drastically changed their dietary habits through globalization and urbanization. They used to consume sago palm, their staple food, along with berries, wild boars, and other wild animals. Nowadays, the consumption of fat and processed foods has increased, and overweight has become an issue among periurban Punan women.

Micronutrient deficiencies, called "hidden hunger," remain a public health issue among certain populations. A recent study suggests that nonpregnant women are at greater risk of clinical vitamin A deficiency, such as night blindness, in families that spend more on rice and less on animal and plant-based foods. Prevention of iodine deficiency continues to be a challenge in the country, where fortification of salt with iodine has not always been successful in some areas of the country. Moreover, the recent food price increase has affected the nutritional status of people in Indonesia. The cost of staple soybean-based products such as tofu and tempeh rose by about 50 percent in 2008. Child malnutrition, including hidden hunger, is on the rise.

Although fat consumption has increased slightly, there is a movement to maintain the traditional diet in Indonesia rather than adopting highly processed global or fast foods. A recent study of contemporary Minangkabau food culture in West Sumatra suggests that their traditional use of coconut may encourage the consumption of fish and vegetables, and, therefore, a well-balanced diet.

Keiko Goto

Further Reading

Campbell, A. A., A. Thorne-Lyman, K. Sun, S. de Pee, K. Kraemer, R. Moench-Pfanner, M. Sari, N. Akhter, M. W. Bloem, and R. D. Semba. "Indonesian Women of Childbearing Age Are at Greater Risk of Clinical Vitamin A Deficiency in Families That Spend More on Rice and Less on Fruits/Vegetables and Animal-Based Foods." *Nutrition Research* 29, No. 2 (2009): 75–81.

Dounias, E., A. Selzner, M. Koizumi, and P. Levang. "From Sago to Rice, from Forest to Town: The Consequences of Sedentarization for the Nutritional Ecology of Punan Former Hunter-Gatherers of Borneo." *Food and Nutrition Bulletin* 28, No. 2 (2007): S294–S302.

Hartini, T. N., R. S. Padmawati, L. Lindholm, A. Surjono, and A. Winkvist. "The Importance of Eating Rice: Changing Food Habits among Pregnant Indonesian Women during the Economic Crisis." *Social Science Medicine* 61, No. 1 (2005): 199–210.

Japan

Population: 127,253,075 (July 2013 est.)
Population Rank: 10th
Population Growth Rate: –0.1% (2013 est.)
Life Expectancy at Birth: 84.19 years (2013 est.)
Health Expenditures: 9.3% of GDP (2011)
People with Access to Safe Drinking Water: 100% of population (2010 est.)
Average Daily Caloric Consumption: 2,810
Adult Obesity Rate: 5% (2008)
Underweight Children under Age 5: Unknown or Negligible

Most Japanese recognize that the key to healthy life can be found in two things: exercise and diet. The Japanese diet as a whole is apparently, with some reservations, extremely healthy. Scientific evidence is emerging that certain foods—kombu and nori, tea, shiitake mushrooms—have health benefits above and beyond their caloric value. The evidence is clear, if nothing else, in the actuarial tables. Notwithstanding the stresses of living in modern Japan, the Japanese consistently come at the head of the life-expectancy tables. Some of the features of Japanese cuisine that have a positive effect on health include the following:

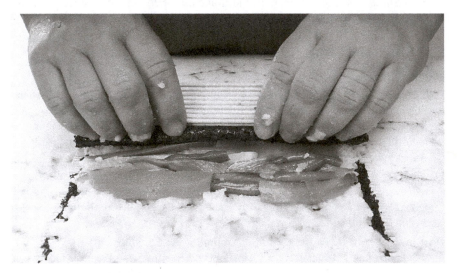

A Japanese chef prepares a sushi roll. (Dobri Dobrinov/iStockphoto.com)

A high proportion of vegetables in the diet: Traditional side dishes are largely based on lightly cooked vegetables: blanching, light steaming, and quick cooking in preference to heavy frying or long stewing. Thus, both caloric value and vitamins are maintained, and more roughage persists in the diet.

Low fat consumption: On the whole Japanese prefer to simmer or grill foods. Deep-frying, though available, is only one of a range of food-preparation methods.

High fish consumption: Japanese have traditionally consumed fatty fish, leading to an increase in high-density lipoprotein (HDL) cholesterol and a decrease in low-density lipoprotein (LDL) cholesterol. Seaweed—lavers, kelps, and true seaweed—which Japanese consume on a regular basis, has beneficial properties, apparently including anticarcinogenic abilities.

Freshness: The Japanese insistence, on the whole, on consuming fresh food, or at least food that has come as quickly as possible from the producer to the consumer (problems of hygiene and modern mass production aside), probably has beneficial aspects as well.

Small servings: Small portions, and lengthy service of desirable meals, have meant that the diner has the time, the emotional resources, and the leisure to savor each morsel and to digest food properly. Japanese meals, consisting of many small portions, ensure that the digestive process is not being put under stress.

Health-promoting foods: There seems to be substantial evidence of active health promotion by foods as diverse as tea, kelp (kombu), and shiitake mushrooms, among others. Tea—green (unfermented), oolong (semifermented and smoked), and black (fermented) types—is regularly consumed by most Japanese: tea is available at work and school breaks, packed for travelers, and as a part of most meals. There are also strong claims by Japanese scientists that consumption of kelp, both cooked and fresh, may help in suppressing absorption of cancer-inducing chemicals. *Katsuobushi* (dried fermented skipjack tuna) flakes (from which dashi, the stock that is heavily used in Japanese cooking, is brewed) have the property of reducing blood pressure, and some studies have shown that the flakes themselves contain amino acids that act to suppress high blood pressure.

In contrast, there are some negative effects of the Japanese diet. These include the following:

High salt levels: Since salt pickles are a major component of the Japanese diet, along with miso, which is brewed with salt, high rates of stomach cancer and high blood pressure are recurring problems in Japan. The Japanese government has taken those findings seriously and has run several campaigns to reduce salt consumption.

Industrial food: Since the end of World War II, the Japanese populace has been affected by a series of problems such as outbreaks of *E. coli,* contaminated milk, and overconsumption of sugar, which have been traced to industrial processes in food manufacturing. Food manufacture is pervasive, and many Japanese households consume large proportions of ready-made meals and industrially produced food. An indication of the extent of factory-processed food is the Japanese government's authorization of the production of purely artificial food bars. Made by biochemists from chemicals and fermentation, they yield full nutritional value with very little taste.

Refined foodstuffs: Until well into the modern era, few Japanese families ate refined white rice as a staple. The process of polishing the rice removes the husk and the germ, which together provide vitamins and protein available only in brown rice. White rice was a desirable commodity, not necessarily an item of daily consumption. White rice is now commonly available, and refined foods such as fish paste (kamaboko), from which much of the vitamins have been removed, are eaten very frequently.

Sugar: The Japanese have become addicted to sugar, and the consumption of sweets in Japan, notably among children, has increased. High consumption of many sweet foods and candies available to Japanese children has contributed to poor dentition among Japanese as they become adults and has also encouraged obesity, which is currently becoming a problem among Japanese children.

Michael Ashkenazi

Further Reading

Ashkenazi, Michael, and Jeanne Jacob. *Food Culture in Japan.* Westport, CT: Greenwood Press, 2003.

Cwiertka, Katrzynka. *Modern Japanese Cuisine: Food Power and National Identity.* London: Reaktion Books, 2006.

Ishige, Naomichi. *The History and Culture of Japanese Food.* London: Kegan Paul, 2001.

Kazakhstan

Population: 17,736,896 (July 2013 est.)
Population Rank: 61st
Population Growth Rate: 1.2% (2013 est.)

Life Expectancy at Birth: 69.94 years (2013 est.)
Health Expenditures: 3.9% of GDP (2011)
People with Access to Safe Drinking Water: 95% of population (2010 est.)
Average Daily Caloric Consumption: 3,360
Adult Obesity Rate: 23.7% (2008)
Underweight Children under Age 5: 4.9% (2006)

As in other former Soviet states, life expectancy in Kazakhstan improved during President Gorbachev's antialcohol campaign of the mid-1980s, fell sharply beginning in 1992, and then began to improve again after 1997. Compared to other newly independent states, its infant and maternal mortality rates remain relatively high, as are its rates for cancer (especially lung cancer, in line with rising tobacco use) and infectious and parasitic diseases such as tuberculosis and hepatitis. The rate of cardiovascular disease in Kazakhstan is higher than in the rest of the region, due to the high rate of consumption of saturated fatty acids and salt.

In common with other Central Asian countries, the core thinking on diet and health is based on the Galenic humoral theories popularized in the region by ibn Sina's *Canon of Medicine* in the eleventh century. Many Kazakh dietary beliefs continue to center on helping to digest the large amounts of saturated fat in the diet. Green tea, sweets, fresh herbs, and fruit all help with the digestion of protein. Green tea also provides valuable antioxidants and vitamins that are helpful in balancing the animal-product-heavy diet. Nonetheless, vitamins A and C are found to be lacking in many people's diets.

Jane Levi

Further Reading

Akshalova, Bakhytgul. *Kazakh Tradition and Ways.* Almaty, Kazakhstan: Dyke Press, 2002.

Fergus, Michael, with Janar Jandosova. *Kazakhstan Coming of Age.* London: Stacey International, 2003.

Laos People's Democratic Republic

Population: 6,695,166 (July 2013 est.)
Population Rank: 102nd
Population Growth Rate: 1.63% (2013 est.)
Life Expectancy at Birth: 63.14 years (2013 est.)

Health Expenditures: 2.8% of GDP (2011)
People with Access to Safe Drinking Water: 67% of population (2010 est.)
Average Daily Caloric Consumption: 2,230
Adult Obesity Rate: 2.6% (2008)
Underweight Children under Age 5: 31.6% (2006)

Years of war reduced the formerly self-sufficient country to conditions that threatened the diet and health of much of the population. The Lao PDR is now a food-insecure country with high malnutrition rates. Insufficient food consumption, in addition to infection and poor health, is the primary cause of malnutrition. Poor diets can also contribute to other problems such as iron deficiency, vitamin A deficiency (resulting in night blindness), and iodine deficiency (resulting in goiter), a common problem in some regions of the country.

The Lao government, along with United Nations partners, is working toward reducing the high infant and under-five mortality rates, as well as maternal mortality rates and malnutrition. The national prevalence of critical food poverty was around 18 percent, indicating that nearly one in five people did not have enough income to buy the food necessary to meet their daily minimum energy requirements. The upland peoples depend more on natural resources than food purchases, but their wild food sources are increasingly threatened as forests are eroded.

Communities depend on traditional herbal medicines, since few people outside of cities have access to primary health care. Herbal medicines are part of health-maintenance systems, not simply treatments for specific diseases. Herbal medicines can be taken orally in alcohol, water, or rice water; swallowed in pill form; or rubbed on the body. They can also be used for a steam "sauna." Herbal saunas are particularly popular with women. Most striking is the number of products used in each concoction; common ingredients include chilies, red ginger, sesame oil, cottonseed, opium, bark, leaves, roots, and ground snail shells. Spirit doctors and shamans practice in some minority communities.

Penny Van Esterik

Gai Yang (Lao-Style Barbecue Chicken)

1 chicken, split open (or use legs and thighs)
Marinade
1 stalk lemongrass, sliced
3 tbsp coriander roots, minced

Pinch salt
1 tbsp fish sauce
2 tsp white pepper
5 cloves garlic
Coconut milk to moisten paste if necessary

Grind marinade ingredients in a small food processor. Rub into the chicken pieces, and marinate at least 3 hours or overnight in the refrigerator. Grill until bottom side is brown; turn over and grill until juices run clear. Serve with steamed glutinous rice and papaya salad.

Further Reading

Du Pont De Bie, Natacha. *Ant Egg Soup: The Adventures of a Food Tourist in Laos.* London: Hodder and Stoughton, 2004.

Hongthong, Penn. *Simple Laotian Cooking.* New York: Hippocrene Books, 2003.

Van Esterik, Penny. *Food Culture in Southeast Asia.* Westport, CT: Greenwood Press, 2008.

Macau

Population: 583,003 (July 2013 est.)
Population Rank: 169th
Population Growth Rate: 0.85% (2013 est.)
Life Expectancy at Birth: 84.46 years (2013 est.)
Health Expenditures: Unknown
People with Access to Safe Drinking Water: Unknown
Average Daily Caloric Consumption: Unknown
Adult Obesity Rate: Unknown
Underweight Children under Age 5: Unknown or Negligible

Macanese cuisine, while heavily Portuguese in nature and not very vegetable-centric, includes many more vegetables in its repertoire than Portuguese cuisine does. This is probably due to influence from Chinese foodways, in which vegetables play a key role in maintenance of a healthy diet. Indeed, no meal is considered complete unless accompanied by at least one vegetable-centric dish. The local Chinese in turn have taken a cue from the Portuguese table and embraced olive oil in their cooking for its healthful properties.

Cholesterol might be a concern for those who consume Macanese specialties on a regular basis. Lard is still a popular choice for cooking and pastry making. Local desserts such as Portuguese egg tarts (the pastry shell is best made with lard), flans, and custards are derived from Portuguese recipes, which tend to rely on egg yolks. The Macanese love their seafood, and seafood in general can be high in cholesterol, but crab—which is the featured ingredient in Macau's famous curried crab dish—is also picked clean of its greenish hepatopancreas (commonly referred to as the "mustard"). The mustard is considered a delicacy, but toxins such as mercury can accumulate here if the crab is raised in polluted waters and therefore it should be consumed with caution.

One of the more unhealthy Macanese dietary habits—the heavy consumption of carbohydrates—can be considered a curious side effect of being influenced by so many cuisines. Minchi, for example, is a popular home-style dish of minced meat with fried diced potatoes that is eaten over rice, often served with a side of bread.

In terms of how the general Macanese population eats, whether Chinese, Portuguese, Macanese, or expatriate, Macau has its share of dietary concerns arising from the increased consumption of processed, junk, and fast foods. Local public health authorities are trying to raise awareness of the risks associated with overconsumption of these foods and promote healthier alternatives.

Karen Lau Taylor

Further Reading

Cheung, Sidney C. H., and Chee Beng Tan, eds. *Food and Foodways in Asia: Resource, Tradition, and Cooking.* London: Routledge, 2007.

Jackson, Annabel. *Taste of Macau: Portuguese Cuisine on the China Coast.* New York: Hippocrene Books, 2004.

Malaysia

Population: 29,628,392 (July 2013 est.)
Population Rank: 43rd
Population Growth Rate: 1.51% (2013 est.)
Life Expectancy at Birth: 74.28 years (2013 est.)
Health Expenditures: 3.6% of GDP (2011)
People with Access to Safe Drinking Water: 100% of population (2010 est.)
Average Daily Caloric Consumption: 2,910

Adult Obesity Rate: 14% (2008)
Underweight Children under Age 5: 12.9% (2006)

Malaysian cooking uses numerous local herbs and spices. These herbs have been used for generations, and they contribute to a healthier diet. For example, kaffir lime leaves provide a refreshing taste that is crucial in many local dishes such as soups, curries, and stews. This leaf can act as a digestive aid and cleanses the blood while helping to maintain healthy teeth and gums. Turmeric root is also another important ingredient in food preparation. It has been used for preparing special dishes such as rendang, *gulai lemak* (beef and coconut stew), and *pais ikan* (fish cooked in banana leaves) to provide an exotic taste to the food. Like the root, the leaf also has many health benefits like aiding digestion, fighting bacteria, and cleansing the system. Another important leaf in Malaysian cooking is *daun kesum,* used in making *laksa* (a noodle soup using fish as the base for the soup). At some places in Malaysia, daun kesum is referred to as *daun laksa* or *laksa* leaves. Daun kesum is a member of the mint family. And, finally, screw-pine leaves are long, narrow, dark green leaves from the screw pine, or pandanus tree. The leaves have a sweet perfume and flavor and are often used in Southeast Asian cooking to flavor rice, puddings, and other desserts. The green color from the leaves is extracted and used as a natural food coloring.

The Chinese in Malaysia use a lot of garlic in their cooking. It can be used to treat high cholesterol, parasites, respiratory problems, poor digestion, and low energy. Studies have found that eating garlic regularly helps lower blood pressure, controls blood sugar and blood cholesterol, and boosts the immune system. It has also been found to reduce the risk of esophageal, stomach, and colon cancer.

In Indian cooking, they use a lot of spices that have medical properties and are good for health. Mostly dried herbs such as cumin, coriander, cinnamon, aniseed, and curry leaves are used. The different cooking styles and ingredients used reflect the demographic variation in the land of origin, which is mainly divided into the northern and southern regions. In addition, Indian cuisines are also influenced by religious beliefs as many dishes are meant to be served to the gods.

M. Shahrim Al-Karim and Che Ann Abdul Ghani

Further Reading

Cheung, Sidney C. H., and Chee Beng Tan, eds. *Food and Foodways in Asia: Resource, Tradition, and Cooking*. London: Routledge, 2007.

Van Esterik, Penny. *Food Culture in Southeast Asia.* Westport, CT: Greenwood Press, 2008.

Māori

Prior to Western contact Māori enjoyed relatively good health. A physically active lifestyle, coupled with a nutritious diet, resulted in a strong and vigorous community. Warfare among Māori was common and was a much greater threat to Māori health than famine or disease. Western contact introduced new diseases that became epidemics in Māori communities, and the Māori Wars increased Māori attrition rates and land confiscations. The Māori were relegated to the lower classes during the colonial period, which has had lasting effects on the Māori peoples.

Poor health and diet continue to plague Māori communities. Māori are among the poorest New Zealanders, which directly affects the modern Māori diet. Like the urban poor in most countries, Māori are plied with inexpensive packaged food that offers little nutritional value. Poor diet is then coupled with poor health care. Although health care in New Zealand is free, Māori remain among the most underserviced, especially in rural areas. The traditional Māori diet would be a far wiser choice than the industrialized diet of today.

Kelila Jaffe

Roroi Kūmara

5 kūmara (sweet potatoes), peeled and grated
$1/4$ c brown sugar
$1/4$ c sugar
2 tbsp butter, melted
1 kūmara (sweet potato), sliced

Mix grated kūmara, brown sugar, sugar, and melted butter in a bowl. Place in a lightly greased baking dish and cover with sliced kūmara. Cover with aluminum foil, and bake at 350°F for 1 hour. Serve warm or cold with whipped cream.

Further Reading

Duffie, Mary Katharine. *Through the Eye of a Needle: A Māori Elder Remembers.* New York: Wordsworth, 2000.

Fuller, David. *Māori Food and Cookery*. Auckland, New Zealand: A. H. and A. W. Reed, 1978.

Mongolia

Population: 3,226,516 (July 2013 est.)
Population Rank: 135th
Population Growth Rate: 1.44% (2013 est.)
Life Expectancy at Birth: 68.95 years (2013 est.)
Health Expenditures: 5.3% of GDP (2011)
People with Access to Safe Drinking Water: 82% of population (2010 est.)
Average Daily Caloric Consumption: 2,250
Adult Obesity Rate: 14.4% (2008)
Underweight Children under Age 5: 5.3% (2005)

On the whole, Mongolians, particularly those living a traditional lifestyle, are a robust people. However, conflicting reports and incomplete research that started only after Soviet withdrawal make it difficult to know precisely how healthy the Mongolian diet is. The traditional Mongolian diet is not well balanced, and some deficiencies have been detected in some groups but not as many as one might expect. Mare's milk is high in vitamin C, which compensates largely for the lack of fruits and vegetables in the diet. The vigorous lifestyle, especially in winter, requires a high calorie intake, and only the meat and dairy diet can supply all the calories needed, especially in a country where people are generally too poor to seek other calorie sources. Some research seems to suggest that, after more than 1,000 years of eating the same thing, Mongolians have either adapted or are genetically predisposed to digesting large amounts of protein.

While the traditional diet may not be perfect, the urban diet has introduced a number of new problems. Dental health has worsened. Children in Ulaanbaatar, where sugar is readily available, have far more cavities and dental problems than nomad children, for whom the consumption of hard cheese offers generally good dental health. The World Health Organization notes that cancer, heart disease, and other problems associated with lifestyle change are increasing. While urban diets have more variety, increasing urbanization also leads to a generally more sedentary lifestyle and greater consumption of refined carbohydrates and highly processed foods, including a switch to sugared soft drinks in place of milk. While vegetables are more available, it remains to be seen whether the added vegetables compensate for the loss of vitamin C and calcium from the consumption of abundant mare's milk. The sedentary lifestyle has, not too surprisingly, led to an increase in obesity in urban settings.

As more people are living in close proximity to one another, there is also the issue of safe water and sanitation. Mongolia is turning to its allies and trade partners for aid in establishing water-safety and sanitation practices that are not necessary when one's nearest neighbor is a few dozen miles away.

The biggest threats to health for those who eat the traditional diet are external. Foremost is the *zud* (also occasionally spelled *dzud*). About every 10 years, Mongolia experiences a zud, or dangerously colder winter than usual. The long winter is normally cold, with January temperatures averaging minus 20 degrees Fahrenheit (minus 30 degrees Celsius). Mongolians and their animals easily survive these ordinary freezes, but a zud takes the temperature much lower or brings a combination of factors, such as heavy snow or a layer of ice, which keep the animals from eating. During the winters of 1999/ 2000 and 2000/2001, approximately 6 million head of Mongolian livestock (sheep, goats, horses, camels, yaks) perished in record zuds. When animals die, people often perish as well, for lack of food. These last two disastrous cold spells threatened the health and food security of approximately 40 percent of Mongolia's population.

Another external threat is marmot hunting. Marmots may be a favored food, but they are rodents—flea-bearing rodents that often have bubonic plague. As a result, there are a few deaths from the plague each summer, usually after marmot-hunting season.

Cynthia Clampitt

Guriltai Shol (Mutton Soup with Noodles)

Traditional Mongolians would make the noodles from scratch as well— simply flat noodles made of wheat flour, water, and a little salt, kneaded, rolled thin, and cut by hand—but in the cities, packets of noodles are available for busy urbanites who no longer have the luxury of time but still long for familiar dishes.

1 lb fatty mutton (beef may be substituted)
1 tsp salt
8 c cold water
Meaty soup bones (optional)

2 medium onions, thinly sliced
4 oz packaged noodles (¾ in. wide)

Cut the meat into strips, as if you were preparing it for a stir-fry dish. Put the meat and 1 tsp salt into the water. (If using soup bones, to create a heartier broth add them to the water, too.) Boil until the meat is thoroughly cooked and water has become a light broth (about 45 minutes), skimming if scum forms. If you used bones, remove them from the broth after the meat is cooked. Then add the onion and noodles, and continue to boil until noodles are done. Taste for seasoning, and add salt if necessary. Soup is ready to serve once the noodles are cooked.

Further Reading

Blundun, Jane, *Mongolia.* 2nd ed. Guilford, CT: Globe Pequot, 2008.

Hudgins, Sharon. "Raw Liver, Singed Sheep's Head, and Boiled Stomach Pudding: Encounters with Traditional Buriat Cuisine."*Sibirica* 3, No. 2 (2003): 131–52.

Thayer, Helen. *Walking the Gobi.* Seattle: Mountaineers Books, 2007.

Nepal

Population: 30,430,267 (July 2013 est.)
Population Rank: 41st
Population Growth Rate: 1.81% (2013 est.)
Life Expectancy at Birth: 66.86 years (2013 est.)
Health Expenditures: 5.4% of GDP (2011)
People with Access to Safe Drinking Water: 89% of population (2010 est.)
Average Daily Caloric Consumption: 2,350
Adult Obesity Rate: 1.4% (2008)
Underweight Children under Age 5: 29.1% (2011)

Because medical resources are limited, especially in remote areas, many Nepalis have recourse to traditional systems of medicine, including Ayurveda, the ancient Indian system of medicine, and Amchi, a Tibetan healing practice. There are an estimated 400,000 practitioners of traditional medicine in Nepal. Both systems rely on the use of local herbs (*jadibuti*) to treat illnesses, and the harvesting of these herbs is a source of income for farmers. In Ayurveda food plays an essential role in preventing and curing illnesses.

It is based on the principle that disease is caused by an imbalance of humors (*doshas*) in the body that can be restored by eating the appropriate foods prescribed by an Ayurvedic physician.

Colleen Taylor Sen

Further Reading

Majupuria, Indra. *Joys of Nepalese Cooking*. Gwalior, India: S. Devi, 1982.

Pathak, Jyoti. *Taste of Nepal*. New York: Hippocrene Books, 2007.

Pakistan

Population: 193,238,868 (July 2013 est.)
Population Rank: 6th
Population Growth Rate: 1.52% (2013 est.)
Life Expectancy at Birth: 66.71 years (2013 est.)
Health Expenditures: 2.5% of GDP (2011)
People with Access to Safe Drinking Water: 92% of population (2010 est.)
Average Daily Caloric Consumption: 2,250
Adult Obesity Rate: 5.5% (2008)
Underweight Children under Age 5: 30.9% (2011)

The Unani system of medicine (Unani tibbia) was introduced into the subcontinent by the Muslim conquerors in the fourteenth century and is adhered to by many Pakistanis. The theoretical framework is derived from the writings of the Greek physicians Hippocrates (460–377 BCE) and Galen (died ca. 200 CE) via the Muslim physician ibn Sina (Avicenna, ca. 980–1037). The Arabic word *Unan* derives from Ionian, the west coast of Turkey, which was at the time part of the Greek world. Unani practitioners are called *hakims*.

Unani medicine is based on the humoral theory of Greek medicine, which assumes the presence of four humors in the body: blood, phlegm, yellow bile, and black bile. Every person is born with a unique humoral constitution, which represents his or her healthy state and determines his or her personality. When the amounts of the humors are changed and thrown out of balance with each other, it leads to disease. Restoring the quality and balance of humors is the goal of treatment, using the body's natural power of self-preservation and adjustment.

Digestion plays a central role in the Unani system. Certain foods can cause indigestion and are to be avoided: those that putrefy quickly (milk and fresh

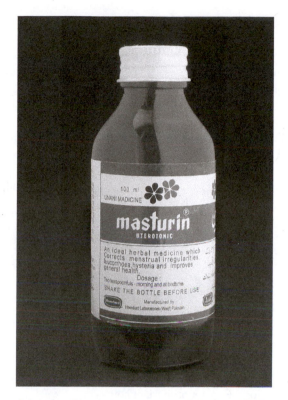

A bottle of herbal medicine used in Unani Tibb,
a traditional healing practice followed by many
Pakistanis. (SSPL/Getty Images)

fish), those that take time to digest (such as beef), stale foods, spices and chilies, alcohol, strong tea, coffee, and oily food. However, any food is acceptable in moderation. Aids to digestion include drinks made from *ajwain* seeds, mint, and fennel and coriander seeds; pomegranate juice; and other herbs and spices.

When a disease is advanced, treatment often begins with a total fast, which gives the patient's system a chance to rest, or with the restriction of food. A liquid diet consisting of fruit juices or soups made from meat or vegetables is prescribed for digestive failure. A semisolid diet comprising yogurt or *khichri* (boiled rice and lentils) is recommended in the case of poor or incomplete digestion.

People are also advised to eat foods that have the opposite quality to their distemper. A person who has too much of the sanguine humor, which leads to increased heat, should eat cold food such as barley water or fish and take cooling herbs; if there is a thinning of the sanguine humor, warm and dry foods are prescribed. For diabetes, bitter and astringent foods are prescribed, such as bitter gourd juice. Weaknesses of specific organs are corrected by eating the same organ of an animal.

Colleen Taylor Sen

Further Reading

Nicholson, Louise. *The Festive Food of India and Pakistan.* London: Kyle Cathie, 2006.

Saiyidain, K. G. *Muslim Cooking of Pakistan.* Lahore, Pakistan: Sheikh Muhammad Ashraf, 2001.

Papua New Guinea

Population: 6,431,902 (July 2013 est.)
Population Rank: 105th
Population Growth Rate: 1.89% (2013 est.)
Life Expectancy at Birth: 66.66 years (2013 est.)
Health Expenditures: 4.3% of GDP (2011)
People with Access to Safe Drinking Water: 40% of population (2010 est.)
Average Daily Caloric Consumption: Unknown
Adult Obesity Rate: 16.2% (2008)
Underweight Children under Age 5: 18.1% (2005)

Papua New Guineans have been interacting with outsiders—missionaries, colonialists, and anthropologists—from as early as 200 years ago to as recently as 60 years ago, but it is only in the last 30 years that most rural villagers have had easier access to imported processed foods. In the past decade, these foods have become an integral part of the PNG diet, with some imported foodstuffs eaten on almost a daily basis. Canned tuna and mackerel, corned beef, and other meat products are now processed in PNG, while other protein sources, such as lamb flaps or turkey tails (Gewertz and Errington 2009), are imported from Australia and New Zealand. Processed imported foods most desired by villagers include white rice, white flour, white sugar, cooking oil, tea, coffee, various biscuits, cookies, and sweet treats. Children in particular desire candy, potato chips, puffed cheese treats, and carbonated soft drinks. None of these foods is particularly nutritious, most are empty calories, and all must be purchased; thus, people need to find a way to make money.

Most recently, the Bariai have exploited the various species of echino-derms, or bêche-de-mer or sea cucumber (B: *anwe*), a traditional foodstuff that was boiled for a long time to make them soft enough to get one's teeth into. For the past few years, women have been collecting and drying bêche-de-mer on a daily basis for sale to visiting buyers, who sell the product to buyers from China, Japan, Hong Kong, and Indonesia. By 2009, bêche-de-mer species had become quite scarce. Bariai women expressed concern that the supply would soon be gone; however, they are reluctant to curtail collect-ing sea cucumbers as these are an exceptionally lucrative income source. Women use money earned from bêche-de-mer sales to pay school and medi-cal fees and buy the imported foods and other goods that were once consid-ered luxury items but have become necessities.

Many villagers in West New Britain, if offered the choice, would prefer canned fish or meat to fresh fish from the sea. Indeed, rice, fried flour, tea or coffee overly sweetened with sugar, canned corned beef, and fish have become especially necessary ingredients for ceremonial feasts. Even with the availability of taro, sweet potatoes, cassava, and sago flour, ceremonies are often put off because no one has money to buy rice, sugar, and tea. The growing need for and consumption of processed foods throughout PNG is beginning to create health problems. When the local Bariai aid-post attendant traveled from village to village for his well-baby clinic, he also lectured the women about diseases associated with eating processed foods (obesity, diabe-tes, heart disease). He tried to impress on the women the importance of grow-ing and eating traditional foods and the sustainability of their lifestyle based on subsistence horticulture. As the need for a cash economy increases and people live off money rather than their gardens and environment, the need to purchase processed and imported foods will increase. The many imported foods that have become an increasingly central part of their diet are an impor-tant issue in food and nutrition studies since these are foods with empty calories and an unhealthy source of sugar, fat, and salt. Obesity, heart disease, and diabetes have become critical health issues in PNG, and there is a move-ment to encourage people to eat local foods grown in their gardens.

Naomi M. McPherson

Further Reading

Ballard, Chris, Paula Brown, R. Michael Bourke, and Tracy Howard. *The Sweet Potato in Oceania: A Reappraisal.* Oceania Monograph 56. Sydney, Australia: University of Sydney. 2005

Gewertz, Deborah, and Fred Errington. *Cheap Meat: The Global Omnivore's Dilemma in the Pacific Islands.* Berkeley: University of California Press, 2009.

Philippines

Population: 105,720,644 (July 2013 est.)
Population Rank: 12th
Population Growth Rate: 1.84% (2013 est.)
Life Expectancy at Birth: 72.21 years (2013 est.)
Health Expenditures: 4.1% of GDP (2011)
People with Access to Safe Drinking Water: 92% of population (2010 est.)
Average Daily Caloric Consumption: 2,520
Adult Obesity Rate: 6.3% (2008)
Underweight Children under Age 5: 20.7% (2008)

The basic Filipino diet conforms to the tenets of what is universally recognized as healthy eating—rice and tubers are high in carbohydrates, fish is an excellent source of protein and omega-3 oils, and vegetables provide necessary vitamins and minerals. While these food groups remain the basis of the Filipino diet, there have been significant changes in dietary patterns over the years, resulting in obesity and increased incidences of serious diseases.

Filipinos are now eating copious amounts of processed foods (including meats, instant noodles, chips, and baked goods) and drinking more soda.

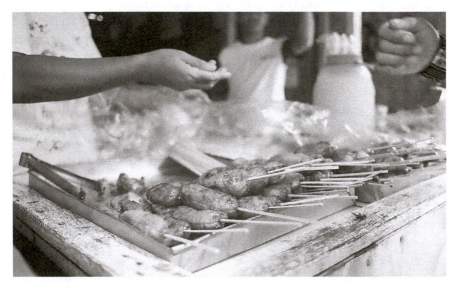

A street vendor sells fried bananas in the Philippines. (Mtkang/Dreamstime.com)

Prices of some processed foods have become even more affordable to the average Filipino than prices of fruits and vegetables. The consumption of fruits and vegetables including roots and tubers has decreased, while consumption of animal-based foods, as well as foods high in sugar, fats, and oils, has increased. Instant noodles are overwhelmingly popular, a major source of empty calories. Many Filipinos are increasingly dependent on street food not just for snacking but for their major meals as well. Most street foods are full of calories, fat, and cholesterol but are highly patronized because of their accessibility, low cost, and ability to fill one up. Restaurant fast foods are now a fixture in the everyday Filipino diet. The incidence of coronary diseases has vastly increased and is associated with the changes in dietary trends in the country. Heart disease is now among the leading causes of adult mortality in the country, alongside tuberculosis, pneumonia, and cancer. Adult obesity continues to rise.

Widespread and fast-growing urbanization, globalization (as evident in the rise of food imports and preference for fast foods), and easier access to technology (cell phones, computers, videos) have all contributed to the significant changes in the Filipino's food-consumption habits. The increased preference for Western foods is a development that has reached even the remotest areas in the country.

With all these changes in the Filipino diet, some things have remained constant. Many Filipinos still turn to the practice of alternative folk medicine by using plants, herbs, vegetables, and other foods to cure common ailments and diseases. Some of these plants and herbs are being manufactured commercially into capsules, powders, and other easily digestible forms. The ampalaya, or bitter melon, widely eaten in the country, is now available in teabag form, and it is being promoted as a treatment for a certain type of diabetes. It is also used for treating cough, liver problems, and sterility. The roots of the *banaba*, a flowering tree, are used for various stomach ailments, and its leaves and flowers for fevers and as a diuretic.

Maria "Ging" Gutierrez Steinberg

Further Reading

Besa, Amy, and Romy Dorotan. *Memories of Philippine Kitchens: Stories and Recipes from Far and Near.* New York: Stewart, Tabori & Chang, 2006.

Fernandez, Doreen G. "Culture Ingested: Notes on the Indigenization of Philippine Food." *Gastronomica: The Journal of Food and Culture* 3, No. 1 (2003): 61–71.

Rodell, Paul. *Culture and Customs of the Philippines.* Westport, CT: Greenwood Press, 2002.

Singapore

Population: 5,460,302 (July 2013 est.)
Population Rank: 115th
Population Growth Rate: 1.96% (2013 est.)
Life Expectancy at Birth: 84.07 years (2013 est.)
Health Expenditures: 4.6% of GDP (2011)
People with Access to Safe Drinking Water: 100% of population (2010 est.)
Average Daily Caloric Consumption: Unknown
Adult Obesity Rate: 7.1% (2008)
Underweight Children under Age 5: 3.3% (2000)

Singapore has an enviable world-class health care system. Despite the culinary focus of the culture, the population has not been beset by the problems of widespread obesity, diabetes, heart disease, and so forth. That said, the government takes an active role in preventative campaigning. In the "Healthy Choices" campaign, for example, Singaporeans are encouraged to select foods that are less rich and lower in fat and to eat coconut-based dishes in moderation because of the high levels of saturated fat. Stalls at hawker markets will display government signs about types of oils, indicating that a "healthy choice" can be made at their stall. Largely, Singaporeans are quite health conscious.

While traditional medical practitioners play a role in Singaporean health care, people are more likely to consult these specialists for minor matters, especially relating to the skin and stress. Additionally, the medicinal properties of food are widely respected by members of the three major ethnic groups, and people will alter their food choices in line with, for example, Chinese medical practices. There are a range of restaurants that cater to these needs. It is possible, for example, to order soups with specific herbs or ones that are prescribed for specific conditions.

All three major ethnic groups in Singapore follow specific dietary practices for pregnancy and the period following birth. The month or so after birth is referred to as the confinement period, which was traditionally characterized by a specific diet and the assistance of a confinement specialist who would cook the required foods and help the mother with the new baby. During this period the mother would not leave the home, hence confinement. Confinement diets are continually evolving and will both prohibit some foods and prescribe others. Today, many Singaporean women follow some of the practices of confinement, especially the confinement diet, and middle-class women still often employ a confinement specialist.

There are significant similarities between Chinese, Malay, and Indian confinement practices, but there are also some important variations. The Chinese confinement diet aims to enhance immunity and to help women regain physical strength. Restrictions include discouraging eating cold food. Cold in this context means both temperature and temperament. It is believed that cold foods can harm the spleen because they retard the discharge of toxins. Foods that are considered cold include some meats and seafoods (especially snails, clams, and oysters), certain fruits (including pomelo, star fruit, and watermelon), a range of vegetables (mushrooms, bitter gourd, water spinach, bamboo shoots), and other items such as seaweed and soy sauce.

Malay mothers in confinement are discouraged from eating spicy food, foods cooked with coconut milk, shellfish, and eggs. Their confinement diet emphasizes soft food, especially soups, often served with rice, as well as noodle dishes. Indian confinement diets also have restrictions and a focus on the role of food as medicinal. Additionally, certain foods are encouraged as aiding bodily functions—for example, brown sugar to expel blood from the uterus or toasted garlic to increase lactation. In all three traditions, women are encouraged to drink warm rather than cold water.

Nicole Tarulevicz

Kaya

Kaya is a jam made with coconut and egg. Its method and qualities are similar to that of lemon curd, only with coconut and pandan (screw pine)-leaf flavoring. As with other jams, kaya is typically spread on toast and is eaten both at breakfast and as a snack. Traditionally kaya is made only with fresh coconuts, but it is possible to make a version with strained coconut milk. To make strained coconut milk, place a piece of muslin in a large sieve, pour a can of coconut cream into the sieve, and leave to drain for an hour.

2 c granulated sugar, if possible caster sugar
4 eggs, lightly beaten
1/2 c thick coconut flesh and milk, from 1 grated coconut
2 pandan (screw pine) leaves, fresh if possible

Place the sugar in a wok (or large saucepan), and slowly heat it, stirring regularly, until the sugar is golden brown. (Do not substitute brown sugar.) When it has become golden, remove the pan from the heat. Once the sugar has cooled a little, transfer it to a large bowl, and add the eggs, one at a time, stirring as you go, and then add the coconut. Beat until the sugar has dissolved. Pour into a pan, and add pandan leaves. On low heat, stir the mixture until it starts to thicken (to test for thickness, place some of the mixture on the back of your spoon and run your finger through it—if it stays separate, then it is ready). Allow the kaya to cool a little before you put it in jars—this gives the pandan leaves extra time to flavor the jam. Remove the leaves just before sealing the jars. Traditionally, this mixture is not refrigerated, but it can be stored in the fridge.

Further Reading

Hutton, Wendy. *The Food of Singapore: Authentic Recipes from the Manhattan of the East.* Singapore: Periplus, 1994.

Oon, Violet. *A Singapore Family Cookbook.* Singapore: Pen International, 1998.

Oon, Violet. *Timeless Recipes: Tasty Singapore.* Singapore: International Enterprise Singapore, 2007.

South Korea

Population: 48,955,203 (July 2013 est.)
Population Rank: 25th
Population Growth Rate: 0.18% (2013 est.)
Life Expectancy at Birth: 79.55 years (2013 est.)
Health Expenditures: 7.2% of GDP (2011)
People with Access to Safe Drinking Water: 98% of population (2010 est.)
Average Daily Caloric Consumption: 3,070
Adult Obesity Rate: 7.7% (2008)
Underweight Children under Age 5: Unknown or Negligible

Taoism was introduced into Korea in the seventh century. The first Taoist temple was built in the twelfth century and was occupied by 11 Korean Taoist monks. However, Taoism never developed into an organization of believers or as a distinct branch of thought on the peninsula. Evidence indicates that elements of Taoism were integrated into shamanism and Buddhism. The national flag of South Korea has the yin-yang symbol in the center and an I Ching trigram at each corner.

Traditional Korean medicine, *hanbang,* is based on the concepts of *chi, eum-yang* (yin and yang), and the five elements: wood, fire, earth, metal, and water. Concepts borrowed from Taoism were translated into Korean ethnomedicine and continue to evolve. Hanbang has a long contiguous history on the peninsula going back thousands of years.

Historically, hanbang had support from various royal dynasties and continued support from postwar governments. Aspects of it permeate Korean culture and persist even in diaspora societies, including among foreign-born Koreans, regardless of educational level and understanding of modern medicine. It is not considered an alternative medicine. Koreans tend to use hanbang remedies for preventative care, for strengthening the immune system, and for detoxification, general weakness, or chronic conditions, while they use Western medicine for acute problems. There is a cultural tendency toward syncretism; the two approaches are viewed as complementary, not contradictory. Hanbang also places importance on proper eating habits. Orally ingested remedies are not just in the form of herbal teas and tonics; food is also medicine.

Modernization has only made hanbang even more popular. It was always a part of Korean spa culture with hot herbal dips, aromatherapy rooms, and salt-bed treatments. More recently, hanbang herbs have been integrated into toiletries and expensive skin-care products. Marketing campaigns incorporate themes of nostalgia as the "natural approach of our ancestors."

Buddhism influenced virtually every aspect of Korean culture. Wonhyo (617–86), a Buddhist monk and great scholar, took Buddhism out of the exclusive realm of the ruling elites and aristocracy. He chose to travel the countryside, spreading Buddhism as penance after siring a son with a Silla princess. Pure-land Buddhism and meditative Buddhism had the greatest impact on Korean religious beliefs. Chinese Ch'an Buddhism was introduced into Korea in the seventh century, where it became interpreted as Son; almost 500 years later it would become Zen in Japan. Son Buddhism is the dominant form of Buddhism in Korea today.

Mahayana monks developed strictly vegetarian temple food. Temple cooking utilizes vegetables and herbs harvested in the mountains. This aspect of temple cooking probably influenced the Korean tendency to make kimchi out of virtually any vegetable. "Hot" vegetables such as garlic, green onion, rocambole (a kind of garlic), and leeks are not used. Temple kimchis do not include salted or fermented fish. The main seasonings are salt, soy sauce, red chili powder, ginger, and sesame seeds. Pine nuts and perilla leaves are used as thickeners. Some temples are renowned for specific types of kimchi.

Susan Ji-Young Park

Further Reading

Lee, Cecilia Hae-Jin. *Quick and Easy Korean Cooking.* San Francisco: Chronicle Books, 2009.

Pettid, Michael J. *Korean Cuisine: An Illustrated History.* London: Reaktion Books, 2008.

Sri Lanka

Population: 21,675,648 (July 2013 est.)

Population Rank: 57th

Population Growth Rate: 0.89% (2013 est.)

Average Daily Caloric Consumption:

Life Expectancy at Birth: 76.15 years (2013 est.)

Health Expenditures: 3.4% of GDP (2011)

People with Access to Safe Drinking Water: 91% of population (2010 est.)

Average Daily Caloric Consumption: 2,390

Adult Obesity Rate: 5.1% (2008)

Underweight Children under Age 5: 21.6% (2009)

Ayurveda, an ancient medicinal system that views the five elements (air, earth, light, water, ether) as connected with the five senses and an individual's biological, psychological, and physiological life forces (*doshas*), is popular in Sri Lanka. The premise is that when doshas are out of balance, disease and illness may prevail. Almost all foods are classified into a "hot" or "cold" framework, whereby over- or underconsumption may contribute to health issues.

Herbs, roots, spices, and dietary changes are often prescribed to address unbalanced doshas. For example, when consumed in moderation, tea is believed to have medicinal properties, ranging from improved digestion to prevention of heart disease.*Gotu kola,* another leafy green plant commonly used in Sri Lankan dishes (*mallung*), is also believed to possess health benefits as a diuretic and mild anti-inflammatory and antibacterial, among other functions.

Mary Gee

Further Reading

Dassanayaka, Channa. *Sri Lankan Flavours: A Journey through the Island's Food and Culture.* Prahran, Australia: Hardie Grant Books, 2003.

Kuruvita, Peter. *Serendip: My Sri Lankan Kitchen.* Sydney, Australia: Murdoch Books, 2009.

Seneviratne, Suharshini. *Exotic Tastes of Sri Lanka.* New York: Hippocrene Book, 2003.

Thailand

Population: 67,448,120 (July 2013 est.)
Population Rank: 20th
Population Growth Rate: 0.52% (2013 est.)
Life Expectancy at Birth: 74.05 years (2013 est.)
Health Expenditures: 4.1% of GDP (2011)
People with Access to Safe Drinking Water: 96% of population
Average Daily Caloric Consumption: 2,530
Adult Obesity Rate: 8.8% (2008)
Underweight Children under Age 5: 7% (2006)

Thailand imported from India some of the ideas about the cooling and heating properties of food and how food affects individuals at certain stages of their life cycle. But since Thailand did not import the South Asian system of castes and subcastes, the heating and cooling properties of food and people had no connotation of purity and pollution; as a result, everyone could eat together.

In the Theravada Buddhist communities of Thailand, some monks, particularly forest monks who reside alone and practice meditation, gain reputations for their skills in healing through herbal and spiritual methods. In the past when villagers might not have had access to any health services, monks were honored as valuable healers who helped reduce suffering out of loving-kindness, free of charge. Ritual speech, words spoken over medicinal mixtures, can be called on in cures. Whether efficacy can be attributed to the placebo effect, or the peace of mind that comes from practicing morality, is not of great concern, particularly in households where no other remedies are available. Spiritual healing is particularly important in palliative care, treating chronic diseases, and when illnesses have a mental health component. Midwives, specialists in traditional massage, herbalists, and shamans all contribute their expertise to the varied healing strategies in Thailand, in addition to the sophisticated and effective public health system in the country.

Food-secure countries like Thailand face a difficult set of problems, as their policy makers must deal with problems related to both under- and over-nutrition. This double dilemma is a result of improvements in food supply combined with changes in food habits. Food security and good health care systems in Thailand are reflected in the low infant and under-five mortality rates in 2005: 18 per 1,000 and 21 per 1,000, respectively. A related challenge concerns the complex interactions between malnutrition and HIV/AIDS. For the many people living with HIV/AIDS in Thailand, adequate and healthy food is their most immediate and critical need, as antiretroviral therapy works effectively only for people who are well nourished.

Although Thailand has low rates of malnutrition, some families may still have to deal with both low-birth-weight infants and overweight schoolchildren. In addition to an estimate of 9 percent low-birth-weight infants and 10–15 percent overweight children in primary schools in the country, about half the people in central Thailand and urban areas now have high cholesterol rates. Changes in food habits and food availability are responsible for this modern "toxic food environment," according to media reports in Thailand. Climbing obesity rates are blamed on Western fast-food chains. Problematic foods are identified as those high in salt, sugar, and fat, including instant noodles, deep-fried chicken, pizzas, hamburgers, French fries, doughnuts, cookies, and cakes. These mouth-watering edibles are found everywhere, leading to increasing rates of coronary heart disease, diabetes, hypertension, and, to some extent, cancer. Heart disease and cancer, diseases of the affluent, are now the primary causes of death in Thailand.

Penny Van Esterik

Tom Kha Gai (Coconut Chicken Soup)

4 c stock
4 chicken breasts, sliced
2 pieces galangal, 1 in. long, split or sliced
4 wild lime leaves, deveined and torn
2 pieces crushed lemongrass, about 2 in. long
4 c coconut milk
4 chilies, sliced
4 tbsp fish sauce

Bring the stock to a simmer, and add chicken, galangal, lime leaves, and lemongrass. Cook 10 minutes or until chicken is cooked through. Add coconut milk, chilies, and fish sauce; heat through and serve.

Further Reading

Brissenden, Rosemary. *Southeast Asian Food.* Singapore: Periplus, 2007.

Muntarbhorn, Kanit. *Gastronomy in Asia, Book I.* Bangkok, Thailand: M. T. Press, 2007.

Thompson, David. *Thai Food.* Berkeley, CA: Ten Speed Press, 2002.

Van Esterik, Penny. *Food Culture in Southeast Asia.* Westport, CT: Greenwood Press, 2008.

Tibet

Known as the "science of healing" (*gsowa rigpa*), Tibetan medicine is an ancient practice with strong links to Buddhist philosophy, Ayurvedic traditions from India, Chinese medicine, and various forms of astrology. It involves a series of complicated diagnoses and treatments including acupuncture, pulse and urine analysis, herbal remedies, diet and lifestyle modifications, heat therapy, and the like. Tibetan medicine upholds the belief that the health of the body depends on the health of the mind. All illnesses, therefore, come from the three poisons of desire, hatred, and ignorance. The ignorant state of consciousness is the root of all disease because it gives rise to desire, which in turn breeds hatred.

Tibetan medical theory asserts that the body is composed of three humors —wind, bile, and phlegm—that control all bodily functions and correspond to the five elements found in nature—earth, water, fire, wind, and space. There are numerous subcategories for each humor as well. The key to good health is to maintain a balance of these humors in the body, in the mind, and in relationship to nature. It is believed that individuals have a tendency toward a predominant humor, or a distinct combination thereof, determining a physical disposition and temperament. That is, a person with a bile temperament is prone to bile-related illnesses.

Furthermore, this system classifies all matter as either hot or cold, both in the environment and in the body. The wind humor is associated with air and thus has a cold quality; bile is linked with fire, producing a hot disposition; and phlegm is associated with earth and water and has a cold quality. Since bile is connected to the element of fire, for example, its function in the body might include producing internal body heat and strength and promoting digestion. And a person with a bile humor, or bile-related illness, has a hot disposition.

Foods are either hot or cold as well, playing an important role in overall health. To promote equilibrium of the body, all foods must be consumed in moderation and should correspond to an individual's predisposition. That is, persons with cool temperaments should consume mostly warm foods, and vice versa. Not only is diet a preventative measure for health, it can be used in healing treatments as well. Many Tibetan doctors prescribe diet modifications to improve internal balance. All the major food groups in Tibetan cuisine are categorized in this manner, and the staples of the local diet are considered some of the healthiest foods. Fresh barley flour (tsampa) is considered a cool food and is believed to cure headaches, stomachaches, and fevers (all hot) if cooked as a porridge with milk. Fresh meat is cool, whereas aged meat is warm and thought to strengthen digestion. These classifications do not correspond with the temperature of the foods but rather their constituents. Broadly speaking, Tibetans believe that cooked foods are superior to anything raw.

In the same manner that a proper diet can restore health, poor food habits are believed to destroy it. An improper diet involves the consumption of anything in excess and the combination of foods that do not belong together. Some examples might include hot milk and fruit, hot milk and sour foods, or drinking cold water with heavy, greasy foods.

Jennifer Hostetter

Further Reading

Jacob, Jeanne, and Michael Ashkenazi. "Tibet." In *The World Cookbook for Students.* Volume 5, *Sri Lanka to Zimbabwe,* edited by Jeanne Jacob and Michael Ashkenazi, 77–83.Westport, CT: Greenwood Press, 2007.

Kelly, Elizabeth. *Tibetan Cooking: Recipes for Daily Living, Celebration, and Ceremony.* Ithaca, NY: Snow Lion, 2007.

Wangmo, Tsering, and Zara Houshmand. *The Lhasa Moon Tibetan Cookbook.* Ithaca, NY: Snow Lion, 2007.

Vietnam

Population: 92,477,857 (July 2013 est.)
Population Rank: 14th
Population Growth Rate: 1.03% (2013 est.)
Life Expectancy at Birth: 72.65 years (2013 est.)
Health Expenditures: 6.8% of GDP (2011)
People with Access to Safe Drinking Water: 95% of population (2010 est.)
Average Daily Caloric Consumption: 2,770
Adult Obesity Rate: 1.7% (2008)
Underweight Children under Age 5: 20.2% (2008)

Chinese medicine, called *thuoc bac,* has long been practiced alongside traditional Vietnamese folk remedies, called *thuoc nam.* Tue Tinh, considered the founder of traditional Vietnamese medicine, was a scholar and Buddhist monk of the fourteenth century. He wrote several books that listed hundreds of medical herbs and thousands of recipes for herbal remedies. Today, common home-based cures for colds and pains include massaging with aromatic oils, inhaling steam imbued with healing herbs, and sipping bitter teas and rich broths.

From the 1940s through the 1980s, the country endured severe shortages of food. A drop in livestock numbers after the Vietnam War, combined with devastating floods in 1978 that destroyed 20 percent of the remaining cattle herds, led to a significant decrease in meat consumption. After the United States lifted its economic embargo against the Communist government in 1994, food from around the world began entering the country. Income levels have doubled every few years since 1990, and after decades of severe food shortages, Vietnam has resumed food exports.

While increasing prosperity has improved the diet of the average Vietnamese, the nutritional status of both children and adults remains poor. The country continues to have one of the highest malnutrition rates in Asia, with 22 percent of children under age five considered low in weight for their age and 33 percent of children under age five considered low in height for their age. For adults, the average consumption is 1,850 calories, or one-fifth less than the accepted minimum daily standard of 2,300 calories.

Thy Tran

Further Reading

Nguyen, Andrea Leigh Beisch, and Bruce Cost. *Into the Vietnamese Kitchen: Treasured Foodways, Modern Flavors.* Berkeley, CA: Ten Speed Press, 2006.

Pham, Mai. *Pleasures of the Vietnamese Table.* New York: HarperCollins, 2001.

Trang, Corinne. *Authentic Vietnamese Cooking: Food from a Family Table.* Burlington, VT: Verve, 1999.

Europe

Armenia

Population: 2,974,184 (July 2013 est.)
Population Rank: 138th
Population Growth Rate: 0.14% (2013 est.)
Life Expectancy at Birth: 73.75 years (2013 est.)
Health Expenditures: 4.3% of GDP (2011)
People with Access to Safe Drinking Water: 98% of population (2010 est.)
Average Daily Caloric Consumption: 2,250
Adult Obesity Rate: 24% (2008)
Underweight Children under Age 5: 5.3% (2010)

Armenian food culture is deeply embedded with medical beliefs and prescriptions for good health. In old times, treatment with food was often the only hope for recovery, not just in rural households, but also in towns. The first hospital did not open in Yerevan, the capital of Armenia, until 1890.

Myths about the healthy qualities of herbs are passed from generation to generation. A person who did not know the medicinal and healthful values of herbs and plants was offensively called *angitats,* "ignorant," by Amidovlat Amasiatsi, the fifteenth-century Armenian physician. Mhitar Heratsi, a famous Armenian physician of the twelfth century, mentions in his writings the primacy of food for survival in both the healthy and the sick.

Fruits are rich in vitamins, and doctors prescribe them for people on low-calorie diets. Armenians used many foods not only to prevent illness but also to cure diseases. Jerusalem artichoke, *getnakhndzor,* is a good substitute for potatoes and starches in diabetic diets. It is sold in large bags during August and September and advertised as a natural insulin. The Chinese date (*Ziziphus jujuba*), called *unab* in Armenian, is a medicine for high blood pressure and chronic cough. Hawthorn, *alotch,* is known as a treatment for heart conditions and high blood pressure.

Meat did not figure prominently in the traditional Armenian diet, not only because it was unaffordable to peasants but also because meatless religious fasts were strictly obeyed by the faithful. In the past, fasting was strictly followed in

185

Armenian communities. Devout Armenians abided by the dictates of the Armenian Orthodox religious calendar and not only fasted before major holidays but also kept weekdays as abstention days. Keeping off meat and dairy products for 158 fast days freed up more resources to be given and distributed to the village community on festive days. Feasting was an extreme activity because it was about overindulgence following the periods of hunger, plus the value placed on certain foods was heightened because they were denied for so long.

Rarely do modern Armenians fast as they did in olden times. Some families do make minor changes to their diets, such as replacing butter with oil or showing a preference for kidney beans or herb soup in the period before Easter or Christmas. The modern pattern of overeating at parties and consuming generous portions of meat, when it is available and affordable, harkens back to the ascetic practices of fasting and abstinence followed by heavy feasting in Armenia.

Irina Petrosian

Spas (Yogurt Soup)

1 c korkot wheat (dried or roasted cracked wheat, similar to bulgur)
7 c water
Salt to taste
1 large onion, finely chopped
3 tbsp butter or vegetable oil
1 tbsp fresh mint, finely chopped
1 tbsp cilantro, finely chopped
1 tbsp parsley, finely chopped
2 c plain yogurt
2 eggs, beaten

Combine korkot with water in a saucepan. Bring to a boil, and lower the heat. Add salt to the liquid, and let simmer for about 1 hour. Sauté the chopped onion in butter or oil until it is golden brown. Remove the skillet from the stove, add seasonings to the onions, and mix well. Pour the contents of the skillet into the saucepan when the korkot becomes tender.

Place yogurt in a bowl. Beat with a spoon until it is smooth. Beat in the eggs. Gradually add a little of the hot liquid from the saucepan to the yogurt mixture while continuously stirring to prevent the egg from curdling. After about 2 cups of liquid have been added to the yogurt, pour the mixture back into the saucepan. Stir for a few minutes until the yogurt is blended. Remove from heat. Serve hot or chilled.

Further Reading

Petrosian, Irina, and David Underwood. *Armenian Food: Fact, Fiction and Folklore.* Bloomington, IN: Yerkir, 2006.

Wise, Victoria Jenanyan. *The Armenian Table: More than 165 Treasured Recipes That Bring Together Ancient Flavors and 21st-Century Style.* New York: St. Martin's Press, 2004.

Austria

Population: 8,221,646 (July 2013 est.)
Population Rank: 94th
Population Growth Rate: 0.02% (2013 est.)
Life Expectancy at Birth: 80.04 years (2013 est.)
Health Expenditures: 10.6% of GDP (2011)
People with Access to Safe Drinking Water: 100% of population (2010 est.)
Average Daily Caloric Consumption: 3,760
Adult Obesity Rate: 20.9% (2008)
Underweight Children under Age 5: Unknown or Negligible

An old Austrian epithet advises against eating too much and too late: "Frühstücken wie ein König, zu Mittag essen wie ein Bürger und zu Abend essen wie ein Bettler" (Eat breakfast like a king, lunch like a townsman, and

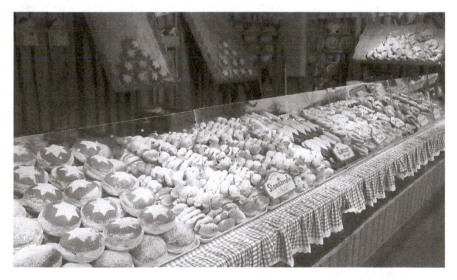

A vast array of pastries being sold in a shop in Vienna, Austria. (iStockPhoto)

dinner like a beggar). During World War II and the subsequent occupation, rationing was severe and Austrians did not have much to eat at all. Following the war, sugar, butter, and other goods became available, and some Austrians overcompensated for their wartime deprivation. The national sweet tooth grew with increasingly available and excellent pastries and confections. Although the daily consumption of sugar in Austria remains somewhat higher than in many other European countries, it has declined in recent years.

The Austrian diet today is generally well balanced, although still excessive in carbohydrates and fats in some regions, leading to the development of diabetes, high blood pressure, and heart disease in some people. Austrians in general, however, are very active and healthy. Many Austrians today, particularly younger, better-educated, and health-conscious citizens, enjoy sweets in moderation and engage in activities such as walking, hiking, cycling, skiing, and other cardiovascular exercise in order to maintain their energy intake/output balance. With their high life expectancies, most Austrians live long, productive lives. Many might gladly admit that they also live very well.

Pamela Elder

Further Reading

Bouley, David, Mario Lohniger, and Melissa Clark. *East of Paris—the New Cuisines of Austria and the Danube.* New York: HarperCollins, 2003.

Mayer-Browne, Elisabeth. *Best of Austrian Cuisine.* New York: Hippocrene Books, 2001.

Rodgers, Rick. *Kaffeehaus: Exquisite Desserts from the Classic Cafes of Vienna, Budapest, and Prague.* New York: Clarkson Potter, 2002.

Basque Territory

The increasing popularity of processed convenience foods has made healthy eating more difficult; obesity and the resulting illnesses are increasing among Basques as they are in the rest of Europe. Street markets, a central Basque commercial and social institution, are losing customers to supermarkets. Daily shopping at outdoor markets is exercise; weekly shopping at supermarkets is not. As the traditional roles gradually break down and yield to more European norms, the health problems that beset modern Western societies are tending to increase. While the traditional Basque diet and lifestyle are extremely healthy, it remains to be seen how they will adapt to the pressures and changes of twenty-first-century life.

Peter Barrett

Further Reading

Barrenechea, Teresa. *The Basque Table*. Cambridge, MA: Harvard Common Press, 1998.

Hirigoyen, Gerald. *Pintxos*. Berkeley, CA: Ten Speed Press, 2009.

Belarus

Population: 9,625,888 (July 2013 est.)
Population Rank: 90th
Population Growth Rate: –0.18% (2013 est.)
Life Expectancy at Birth: 71.81 years (2013 est.)
Health Expenditures: 5.3% of GDP (2011)
People with Access to Safe Drinking Water: 100% of population (2010 est.)
Average Daily Caloric Consumption: 3,090
Adult Obesity Rate: 24.3% (2008)
Underweight Children under Age 5: 1.3% (2005)

Food has been seen as medicinal in Belarus. For instance, combinations of vegetable or herb juices with honey and alcohol are common folk remedies for many illnesses. Many medicinal plants were gathered on Kupalle night, as it was believed that their power is then at its peak. These beliefs remain today as well. Major newspapers, books, and calendars contain articles, often submitted by the readers themselves, about various folk remedies. Mint or lime-tree tea is considered helpful for dizziness. A plaster made of hot mashed potato mixed with vodka and honey applied to the chest and back is said to prevent colds and coughs.

Belarusians eat many starchy foods and a lot of fatty pork. In the past, heavy work in the fields made this traditional diet a necessity. In the past, access to fresh herbs and berries from the woods aided Belarusians in obtaining enough vitamins in their diet. Today, most of the population lives in cities and is relatively poor. Belarusians rely on inexpensive foods to provide most of their daily energy intake.

Due to the fairly cold climate they have little access to or inclination to eat more fresh fruit and vegetables out of season, and poor exchange rates prevent their importation. Heavy drinking and smoking, imported from the former Soviet Union, remain serious problems. These factors lead to about half of Belarusians dying in their mid-60s from cardiovascular diseases.

Industrial pollution and remaining radiation from neighboring Ukraine's Chernobyl nuclear disaster in 1986 have tainted some Belarusian farming land, water, and the food supply. The concern about pollution remains strong for many people, who ask farmers about the origins of food in farmers' markets. These concerns are also addressed by the marketing of many food brands as coming from "ecologically pure" sources.

Anton Masterovoy

Further Reading
Bely, A. *The Belarusian Cookbook.* New York: Hippocrene Books, 2009.

Belgium

Population: 10,444,268 (July 2013 est.)
Population Rank: 83rd
Population Growth Rate: 0.05% (2013 est.)
Life Expectancy at Birth: 79.78 years (2013 est.)
Health Expenditures: 10.6% of GDP (2011)
People with Access to Safe Drinking Water: 100% of population (2010 est.)
Average Daily Caloric Consumption: 3,690
Adult Obesity Rate: 22.1% (2008)
Underweight Children under Age 5: Unknown or Negligible

Today, in Belgium, food is on sale 24 hours a day, and most Belgians may eat whatever, whenever, and wherever they want. Compared with the past, this is a drastic change. If the pre–World War II food-related problems are viewed in terms of shortage and imbalance, with lack of calories, vitamins, and protein, leading to loss of weight and strength, edema, anemia, lethargy, and, for children, slow growth, the post-1950 abundance has caused problems of a new kind related to body shape and health: being overweight and obese increases the risk of diabetes, cardiovascular diseases, hypertension and stroke, and some cancers.

Today, 52 percent of the Belgians are considered to have a "normal" weight according to the body mass index (BMI, or the relation between a person's weight and height). The number of obese people, however, is growing slowly but constantly, and about 13 percent of Belgians are considered obese (with a BMI over 30). This worries nutritionists, doctors, and health workers, and public organizations regularly launch information programs aimed at convincing Belgians to move more such as by using the stairs instead of the elevator, while eating less sweet and fat food. Belgians have many ways of trying to lose weight. Slimming products such as laxatives are popular, but starting exercise, or simply more physical effort, is rarely considered. A minority of Belgians call on a physician for help with losing weight, and stomach reduction has gained popularity. However, the most popular way of losing weight is dieting. This takes many forms: eating less in general, eating less sweet and/or fat food, eating more fruit and vegetables, skipping meals, starting to use diet products, and/or following, strictly or loosely, the latest fad in dieting.

Slimming is not necessarily prompted by health concerns but may be purely cosmetic, to attain the ideal body. Slim ideals appeared among the higher social classes in Belgium in the 1920s but spread to all classes in the 1950s. By the end of the 1930s, many cookbooks suggested a reduction in consumption of meat, cheese, and eggs, for both health reasons and slimming. Calories started to rule the lives of thousands of people.

The public authority's influence on what Belgians eat has largely increased in terms of safety monitoring, information, and recommendations. Belgians nowadays eat more safely than ever before, and, above all, they are much more informed about the tiniest food risk, food-safety procedures in supermarkets, organic foods in cafeterias, and dieting schemes. Yet despite the greater sensitivity regarding health and safety of food, recent crises have shown the very feeble trust most people have in the food chain. For some, eating copiously provides the badly needed security in today's uncertain times.

Peter Scholliers

Smoutebollen or Beignets (Doughnut Balls)

1 tbsp yeast
$1/3$ c milk
$12/3$ c flour
1 egg
1 tsp sugar
$1/2$ tsp salt
1 small bottle witbier (white beer, Hoegaerden type)

2 tbsp butter
Oil for deep-frying

Dissolve the yeast in the lukewarm milk, and add the flour, sifting it well. Separate the egg, and add the egg yolk, sugar, salt, and beer to the milk-and-flour mixture; stir well, and add the melted butter. Then, beat the egg white and fold it gently into the dough. Cover the dough, and let rise until its volume has doubled. Keep it out of the cold. Heat the oil to 350°F. Very gently stir the dough, then drop teaspoonfuls of the dough gently into the frying oil and fry until golden brown, which takes about 1 minute. Use a slotted spoon to remove the doughnuts from the fryer, lay on a plate covered with a paper towel to absorb excess oil, and serve with powdered sugar.

Further Reading

Jacobs, Marc, and Jean Fraikin. "Belgium: Endives, Brussels Sprouts and Other Innovations." In *Culinary Cultures of Europe: Identity, Diversity and Dialogue,* edited by Darra Goldstein and Kathrin Merkle, 75–85. Strasbourg, France: Council of Europe Publishing, 2005.

Scholliers, Peter. *Food Culture in Belgium.* Westport, CT: Greenwood Press, 2008.

Van Waerebeek, Ruth, and Maria Robbins. *Everybody Eats Well in Belgium Cookbook.* New York: Workman, 1996.

Bosnia and Herzegovina

Population: 3,875,723 (July 2013 est.)
Population Rank: 128th
Population Growth Rate: –0.1% (2013 est.)
Life Expectancy at Birth: 76.12 years (2013 est.)
Health Expenditures: 10.2% of GDP (2011)
People with Access to Safe Drinking Water: 99% of population (2010 est.)
Average Daily Caloric Consumption: 3,080
Adult Obesity Rate: 26.5% (2008)
Underweight Children under Age 5: 1.6% (2006)

The traditional Bosnian diet is basically healthful. Instead of being fried, for instance, meats are often simmered, and vegetables are cooked in the meat juices. These vegetable and meat one-dish meals are very common. The diet is grain based; bread, whether made of wheat, barley, or corn, is an essential part of nearly every meal, and polenta (*pura*) and buckwheat mush are surviving traditional foods. Meat makes up about 40 percent of the national diet, though in mountain villages the amount may be far less. In villages fresh meat generally is eaten on auspicious occasions but otherwise used sparingly. Milk products are essential to the diet. Soured cultured milk is heavily consumed in urban centers, and whey from churned butter in villages. Bosnians shop regularly at open markets where they buy seasonal fruits and vegetables, which they eat fresh and preserve for winter. Buying local without being particularly conscious about it is a Bosnian tradition.

Yvonne R. Lockwood and William G. Lockwood

Further Reading

Marin, Alma. "The Unbearable Lightness of Wartime Cuisine." *Gastronomica: The Journal of Food and Culture* 5, No. 2 (2005): 27–36.

Tanovic, Nenad. "Bosnia and Hercegovina." In *Culinary Cultures of Europe: Identity, Diversity and Dialogue,* edited by Darra Goldstein and Kathrin Merkle, 87–93. Strasbourg: Council of Europe Publishing, 2005.

Bulgaria

Population: 6,981,642 (July 2013 est.)
Population Rank: 101st
Population Growth Rate: –0.81% (2013 est.)
Life Expectancy at Birth: 74.08 years (2013 est.)
Health Expenditures: 7.6% of GDP (2010)
People with Access to Safe Drinking Water: 100% of population (2010 est.)
Average Daily Caloric Consumption: 2,760
Adult Obesity Rate: 23.7% (2008)
Underweight Children under Age 5: 1.6% (2004)

While herbalism has long held an honored place in Bulgarian home treatment, the economic hardships of the 1990s placed Western prescription medicines beyond the financial reach of many Bulgarians, leading many to look inwardly to traditional methods of medical care once again. For instance, čubrica, summer savory, is said, when rubbed on an insect sting, to soothe

the skin's painful reaction, but it is also used more generally as a pick-me-up, as an expectorant to help clear phlegm in the lungs and sinuses, and as a preventative of diarrhea and reliever of colic and flatulence. Although there has been debate in Bulgarian food culture about whether the onion should be considered a spice, its efficacy is not questioned. Onion is considered to have some medicinal properties and to stimulate the secretion of gastric juices. It appears raw in salads and travels through Bulgarian cookery, appearing in stews, sauces, and preserves. Bulgaria has great resources of mineral waters, most notably the spring-fed water in a number of towns that cluster around Plovdiv: Brasigovo and Hisarja. Used to treat gastrointestinal disorders, such water is also bottled and distributed commercially. Soup also holds a place in the panoply of anecdotal food "cures" in Bulgaria: the tripe soup shkembe chorba reputedly alleviates the gastrointestinal problems associated with hangovers.

Fiona Ross

Further Reading
Davies, Trish. *The Balkan Cookbook: Traditional Cooking from Romania, Bulgaria and the Balkan Countries.* London: Anness, 1999.

Croatia

Population: 4,475,611 (July 2013 est.)
Population Rank: 124th
Population Growth Rate: –0.11% (2013 est.)
Life Expectancy at Birth: 76.2 years (2013 est.)
Health Expenditures: 7.8% of GDP (2010)
People with Access to Safe Drinking Water: 99% of population (2010 est.)
Average Daily Caloric Consumption: 2,990
Adult Obesity Rate: 24.2% (2008)
Underweight Children under Age 5: Unknown or Negligible

Croatia has a long tradition of folk medicine and home remedies, many of which are still adhered to among the highly educated elite. In June 2009, health minister Darko Milinovic surprised his colleagues by saying at a press conference that honey, tea, and lemon along with frequent showers was a cure for swine flu. He retracted that claim almost immediately, but it did reveal a typical belief that a simple good diet promotes health.

Croatia has a long tradition of using herbs such as caraway, juniper, and walnut kernels for intestinal problems; mallow, chamomile, mint, and lemon balm for sore throats and cough; and elderflower to improve circulation. Other remedies have more of a magical aspect, as in the burning of alecost with wormwood and rose petals; supposedly, inhaling the smoke has special healing powers. *Raki,* the grape brandy, is used to make herb infusions and also externally to heal wounds or bruises. Wrapping a sore throat in a towel soaked in *lozovac,* a locally produced brandy, is said to aid in healing.

Still, the best folk remedies in the world are powerless against unhealthy modern dietary practices. Changes in the Croatian diet have had a strong negative effect on coastal Croatians; a study conducted in 2003 showed that the percentage of overweight people among residents of Dalmatia had increased to 54 percent of men and 48 percent of women, and 27 percent of both genders were obese. The authors of the study theorized that this was because the islanders now eat much more meat than their ancestors and have not changed their lifestyle accordingly.

Islanders are still healthier than inland Croats. Cardiovascular disease is the leading cause of death in Croatia, and a study from the Croatian Public Health Institute in 2005 showed that inland Croats were far more likely to suffer a heart attack. A poor diet was cited as a major factor. A 2009 study of multiple sclerosis and cancers in Croatia showed that both diseases were twice as common in the inland areas where the diet is rich in meat and fat and suggested that the high intake of olive oil among coastal residents was protecting them from the same fate. The government has been trying to encourage a return to traditional healthy practices such as increased consumption of fish instead of meat. This includes financing a campaign called *Srdela snack,* encouraging people to eat sardines instead of other fast food. It has been relatively successful, but sardine sandwiches still have not replaced hamburgers and cevapi as the most popular quick meals.

Regardless of their region, Croatians have a very high rate of smoking and consumption of alcohol, and the government is taking steps toward discouraging these unhealthy practices. A tobacco ban in restaurants went into effect in 2009 but has been widely ignored; nevertheless, a study by Euromonitor predicted that this ban, combined with an increase in tobacco taxes, will start to reduce tobacco use. An increase in the tax on hard alcohol went into effect in 2007 but has had little social effect for several reasons. It does not apply to wine and beer, cannot be imposed on the brandy and other liquors that are widely homemade, and, even when it is applicable, is widely avoided. These statistics aside, the general level of health in Croatia is superior to that in most of the other former Yugoslav republics, and the life expectancy of 76 years is not far from the European Union average.

Richard Foss

Further Reading

Evenden, Kate. *A Taste of Croatia*. Ojai, CA: New Oak Press, 2007.

Pavicic, Liliana. *The Best of Croatian Cooking*. New York: Hippocrene International Cookbooks, 2000.

Cyprus

Population: 1,155,403 (July 2013 est.)
Population Rank: 160th
Population Growth Rate: 1.52% (2013 est.)
Life Expectancy at Birth: 78.17 years (2013 est.)

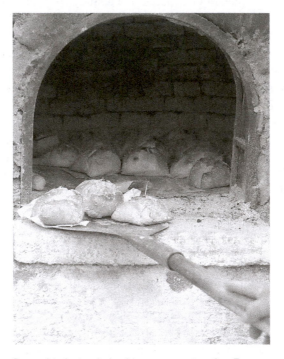

Bourekia being baked in preparation for Easter celebrations in Cyprus. (Shutterstock)

Health Expenditures: 7.4% of GDP (2011)
People with Access to Safe Drinking Water: 100% of population (2010 est.)
Average Daily Caloric Consumption: 3,200
Adult Obesity Rate: 25.5% (2008)
Underweight Children under Age 5: Unknown or Negligible

Traditional Cypriot cuisine is an ideal example of the widely praised Mediterranean diet. Its foundation is a healthful mix of grains, legumes, vegetables, and fruits, with meat and fish eaten sparingly once or twice a week. Holidays and celebrations call for richer, more indulgent foods throughout the island, but they are balanced in both the north and the south by religious days of fasting and abstention, such as Ramadan in the north and Lent in the south.

That pattern is likely to be challenged, however, now that tourism has become an important driver in the country's economy. Today, restaurants supply holiday foods every day of the week to visitors and Cypriots alike. As the Cypriot standard of living rises, this temptation will become increasingly difficult to resist.

Nancy G. Freeman

Further Reading

Sakkadas, Savvas. "Cyprus: Culinary Traditions throughout the Year." In *Culinary Cultures of Europe: Identity, Diversity and Dialogue,* edited by Darra Goldstein and Kathrin Merkle, 119–28. Strasbourg: Council of Europe Publishing, 2005.

Weaver, William Woys. "Bold Flavors, Ancient Roots." *Saveur* 111 (May 2008): 54–65.

Czech Republic

Population: 10,162,921 (July 2013 est.)
Population Rank: 86th
Population Growth Rate: −0.15% (2013 est.)
Life Expectancy at Birth: 77.56 years (2013 est.)
Health Expenditures: 7.4% of GDP (2011)
People with Access to Safe Drinking Water: 100% of population (2010 est.)
Average Daily Caloric Consumption: 3,320
Adult Obesity Rate: 32.7% (2008)
Underweight Children under Age 5: 2% (2007)

Traditional Czech cuisine is heavy in salt and saturated fats. As such, the Czech Republic has one of the highest rates of death due to cardiovascular disease in the developed world. As more awareness is given to health and diet, more and more Czechs are dieting or watching their weight.

To eat dietetically, Czechs increase their consumption of fresh fruits and vegetables. Grapefruit and pineapple are considered "fat eaters" and are popular diet foods eaten at breakfast. This is in contrast to eating foods that have the fat or sugar removed. Cheeses, potato chips, milks, and yogurts are all full fat. It is believed that the fat is more natural in these foods.

Czechs have a long tradition of using spas as a health and wellness resource, both for treatment of chronic medical conditions as well as for relaxing vacations. These spas, mostly located around natural mineral springs, take advantage of mountainous forested areas. These resorts have special spa food with more fresh vegetables and lower-fat meats and fishes. It is not uncommon to go to one for several weeks to a month to recover from an illness.

Brelyn Johnson

Cesnekova Polevka (Garlic Soup)

6 cloves garlic
3 tbsp butter
14 oz chicken stock
1 egg per person
Spring onions, sliced
3 oz semisoft, mild cheese, like Gouda
3 oz ham, diced
1 c hard white bread, diced and fried for croutons

Fry the garlic in butter until aromatic, add stock, and bring to a boil for 10 minutes. Turn the burner to low. Add the egg(s) softly to the pot, and let sit for 5 minutes. Spoon eggs with broth into serving bowls. Add spring onions, cheese, and ham. Add croutons to the soup.

Further Reading

Polvany, Marina. *All along the Danube: Recipes from Germany, Austria, Czechoslovakia, Yugoslavia, Hungary, Romania and Bulgaria.* New York: Hippocrene Books, 1994.

Trnka, Peter. *The Best of Czech Cooking.* New York: Hippocrene Books, 1996.

Denmark

Population: 5,556,452 (July 2013 est.)
Population Rank: 111th
Population Growth Rate: 0.23% (2013 est.)
Life Expectancy at Birth: 78.94 years (2013 est.)
Health Expenditures: 11.2% of GDP (2011)
People with Access to Safe Drinking Water: 100% of population (2010 est.)
Average Daily Caloric Consumption: 3,400
Adult Obesity Rate: 18.2% (2008)
Underweight Children under Age 5: Unknown or Negligible

With an average life expectancy of almost 79 years, low infant-mortality rates, and an HIV prevalence of less than 1 percent, Denmark has a generally healthy population. Cancer is the leading cause of death, followed by heart disease. This good health is thanks in large measure to a highly efficient public health system, partly funded by Denmark's global leadership in diabetes treatment, antibiotics, and psychotropic medication. It is also thanks to a general lifestyle that includes a fair amount of physical activity—cycling is the most common mode of transport, for children and adults alike, and large parts of most cities are reserved for pedestrians. However, in recent decades, Denmark has also experienced increasing numbers of people who are overweight or obese, particularly children. This is most often explained as a result of increased consumption of fast food, sweets, and convenience products.

The country does have a long history of monitoring food and diets in the interests of public health. The first major study of the nutrient values of foods was undertaken by physiologist and pathologist P. L. Panum in the 19th century. Panum's work was developed by a number of scientists over the next century or so, notably Christian Jürgensen (author of the first table of "Common Recommendations for the Healthy and the Ill" in 1888) and Richard Ege, whose 1932 nutrition tables incorporated the then newly discovered vitamins and who continued to publish significant work until the 1970s, when Peder Helms's computerized tables paved the way for the first national Danish Food Composition Database, which published its first official tables in the 1980s. These nutritional databases have been instrumental in compiling dietary recommendations for the Danish population.

The first official food pyramid was launched in 1976 by FDB, a retail cooperative that has been involved in consumer welfare for more than a century. In 1996 they introduced the "S" symbol on supermarket products that were certified as healthy choices (*sundhed* is the Danish word for health). In 2009, following a merger with other Nordic countries, this was replaced by the keyhole symbol that had been introduced in Sweden some years earlier. Criteria for the keyhole include acceptable amounts of fat, sugar, fiber, and salt. Its effectiveness is yet to be measured. As the rest of the world tunes in to not just the gastronomic delights but also the supposed healthfulness of the so-called new Nordic diet with its emphasis on local grains, berries, and fish, it remains to be seen whether Danes themselves will find the fairytale compelling enough to prefer rye bread and herring to a frozen ready-made portion of Moroccan-spiced chicken from the supermarket.

Signe Rousseau

Further Reading

Hahnemann, Trine. *The Scandinavian Cook-book.* Kansas City, MO: Andrews McMeel, 2009.

Halkier, Bente. "Performances and Positionings in Cooking Practices among Danish Women." *Food, Culture and Society* 12, No. 3 (2009): 357–77.

Notaker, Henry. *Food Culture in Scandinavia.* Westport, CT: Greenwood Press, 2008.

Finland

Population: 5,266,114 (July 2013 est.)
Population Rank: 116th
Population Growth Rate: 0.06% (2013 est.)
Life Expectancy at Birth: 79.55 years (2013 est.)
Health Expenditures: 8.9% of GDP (2011)
People with Access to Safe Drinking Water: 100% of population (2010 est.)
Average Daily Caloric Consumption: 3,220
Adult Obesity Rate: 23% (2008)
Underweight Children under Age 5: Unknown or Negligible

Diet and health are important issues in Finnish society and are often mentioned when talking about food. In the 1960s mortality due to heart disease was very high among men, and a major health-promoting project to prevent cardiovascular disease in North Karelia started in the 1970s. It was a big success. Butter, whole milk, and fatty dishes were abandoned in favor of lighter oil-based products, vegetables, and fibers. Still, as in so many Western countries, being overweight is a big problem that causes many health problems such as diabetes. The Development Program for the Prevention and Treatment of Diabetes (DEHKO, 2000–2010) is a national program, the first worldwide to include and implement the prevention of type 2 diabetes. Life has become easier in a way; food is everywhere, and most people do not burn all the calories they take in. Physical work is replaced by sitting still all day long in an office, and people need a lot of information to be able to take care of their health.

Finland is a pioneer developer of health-enhancing foodstuffs. Nutrition research is internationally recognized at a high level, and also many remarkable inventions in functional food development have been made. Probiotics, prebiotics, plant flavonoids, plant sterols, dietary fiber, and more are important ingredients in functional food, seen as a new possibility to promote well-being by using "tailored" foods. Benecol, Xylitol, and Lactobacillius GG are officially approved examples of Finnish food innovations.

Finnish researchers have also pointed out several products that are naturally health enhancing such as rye bread, berries, rapeseed oil, oat products, and buckwheat products. Finnish meat, grain, vegetables, and berries are considered to be very clean. Pollution is limited, and not many insecticides are used compared with many other southern countries because of cold winters and strict regulations. There are also about 4,500 organic farms in Finland, representing 6 percent of all farms. The organic food production has a reliable reputation since the authorities enforce strict regulations throughout the whole organic food chain.

There is an increasing demand for special diet food as well. Many clients in restaurants, patients in hospitals, and students in school need a special diet because of their diseases. High cholesterol, diabetes, celiac disease, and many food allergies have united developers in the food industry and medical scientists to find solutions for dietary needs in society. In fact, Finland has one of the oldest dietary industries in the world.

The reason public authorities focus on nutrition and eating habits is for the prevention and treatment of diseases. The National Nutrition Council in Finland makes statements and recommendations, but Finns wonder about the relationship between food and pleasure and health. In the south of Europe, food and eating are considered to be pleasurable. The Nordic tradition is more spartan; food has for a long time been merely a nutrient, something one needed to survive but not for pleasure. If one is really enjoying a meal, there must be some reason to feel guilty. Something being both healthy and good tasting seems impossible.

Yrsa Lindqvist

Further Reading

Bourret, Joan Liffring-Zug, Jerry Kangas, and Dorothy Crum, eds. *Finnish Touches: Recipes and Traditions.* Iowa City, IA: Pennfield Press, 2002.

Hill, Anja. *The Food and Cooking of Finland.* London: Anness, 2007.

France

Population: 65,951,611 (July 2013 est.)
Population Rank: 21st
Population Growth Rate: 0.47% (2013 est.)
Life Expectancy at Birth: 81.56 years (2013 est.)
Health Expenditures: 11.6% of GDP (2011)
People with Access to Safe Drinking Water: 100% of population (2010 est.)
Average Daily Caloric Consumption: 3,550
Adult Obesity Rate: 18.2% (2008)
Underweight Children under Age 5: Unknown or Negligible

Variety has characterized the French way of eating since the end of World War II. The diet is relatively high in fruits, vegetables, grains, and legumes, in addition to meats, cheeses, and other dairy products. The use of butter fats, animal fats such as lard and goose fat, and vegetable oils used to vary largely by region. At present, the broad preference for cooking with vegetable oils such as sunflower oil stems from their lower prices, on the one hand, and information about health benefits associated with unsaturated vegetable oils and the Mediterranean diet, on the other. Wine was long viewed as a healthful, strengthening beverage and in this sense was perceived as different from distilled alcohols. Despite this perception, rates of alcoholism and diseases such as cirrhosis of the liver were high through the mid-twentieth century. In this nation of wine drinkers, the *crise de foie* (liver crisis) was a classic complaint, extensible to nearly any malaise. The view that wine is healthful has not disappeared, but consumption has declined. Water is the most widely consumed beverage.

The French associate eating the full three-course meal with a sense of well-being and with good health. The structured family meal provides nutritional balance. It conditions daily eating while contributing to the highly valued quality of life. The benefits of eating the full three-course family meal are thought of in a holistic fashion. The American practice of counting calories and weighing portions would seem strange to most French. Rather, eating a broad selection of fresh foods is understood as key to *une bonne nutrition* or *une alimentation saine* (good nutrition, a healthful diet). And variety is precisely what characterizes the full meal with its complement of three or four different dishes.

Beyond nutrition, culinary quality and the appreciation of food are essential to the perception of eating well. Conviviality and social connection to family and friends are equally necessary ingredients. The respite imposed by the slow rhythm of the full meal cannot be discounted. People use the terms *équilibre* (balance), *modération* (moderation), and *plaisir* (enjoyment, pleasure) to name the salient features of eating well, and *harmonieuses* (harmonious) to describe the ensemble of practices that go into eating well. These ideas guide practical aspects of cooking and serving, such as determining the relatively small portion sizes for meal components.

In the past, most health care was given at home, including for severe illnesses. Home cooks and cookbooks had a repertoire of foods for the sick, such as "pectoral" broths to strengthen the lungs. Today, there remains little concept of specific foods appropriate for the ill. Adjustments are made to the diet, such as excluding greens and salads, in favor of plain boiled rice and cooked carrots, until a stomach ailment has passed, or reducing protein on a daily basis in the case of a chronic kidney problem. To improve digestion, people take mineral waters high in magnesium, salads, fresh fruits and vegetables, yogurt, or a drink of pastis (anise liquor).

The general health of the population is relatively good. To be sure, as in other affluent nations, abundance, the modern lifestyle, and agricultural and manufacturing practices create dietary dilemmas. For some, *grignotage* (snacking) replaces or augments the cycle of three daily meals. The sedentary lifestyle combined with an unbalanced diet contributes to rising levels of obesity and diabetes. Pathological behaviors related to eating and having psychological causes, such as anorexia and bulimia, are on the rise. Genetically modified foods and agribusiness practices are perceived as threats to health. Yet other indicators remain quite positive. The life span for women is more than 83 years, the longest in Europe. The national health system, which provides nearly universal access to high-quality medical care, emphasizes prevention. The state, which regulates health care, has stressed intervention, such as removing vending machines from public schools in 2005 to reduce young people's consumption of sugar, salt, and fat as empty calories in junk food. In France, the precautionary, preventive, and interventionist attitude plays a role in maintaining public health, while the shared strong emphasis on food culture enhances *la vie à la française*—the French way of life.

Julia Abramson

Ratatouille (Summer Vegetable Stew)

This is a typical entrée for cooking and eating at home.

7 tbsp olive oil
1 lb zucchini and/or yellow crookneck squash, sliced into rounds
2 green or red peppers, seeded, membranes removed, and sliced
1 eggplant (about 1 lb), cut into 1-in. cubes
1½ c chopped onion
2 tbsp chopped garlic
2 lb tomatoes, halved and seeded
6 sprigs thyme, leaves stripped from the stems
6 tbsp chopped parsley
8 tbsp chopped basil
Salt
Ground black pepper

Heat 2 tablespoons of the olive oil in a large skillet over moderate heat. Sauté the zucchini about 6 minutes until lightly browned. Using a slotted spoon, transfer to a large bowl.

Add 1 tablespoon of oil to the skillet, then sauté the sliced peppers for 5 minutes, and transfer to the bowl.

Add 3 tablespoons of oil to the skillet, then put in the eggplant. Stir to prevent the eggplant from sticking to the pan. Cook until the eggplant is soft, light-colored, and smooth in texture (about 8 or 9 minutes). Add to the bowl with the other vegetables.

Pour the last tablespoon of olive oil to the pan, and sauté the onion and garlic for about 3 minutes, watching carefully to prevent them from browning much. Add the tomatoes, thyme, and half the parsley. Simmer for 10 minutes. Return all the vegetables in the bowl back into the pan with the tomatoes, stir gently to mix, and cook for 10 more minutes. The vegetables should be cooked through and tender but not mushy.

Take the pan off the heat. Stir in the rest of the parsley and the basil. Season with salt and pepper. Serve hot, cold, or at room temperature.

Further Reading

Abramson, Julia. *Food Culture in France*. Westport, CT: Greenwood Press, 2007.

de la Pradelle, Michèle. *Market Day in Provence*. 1996. Translated by Amy Jacobs. Chicago: University of Chicago Press, 2006.

Fischler, Claude, and Estelle Masson. *Manger: Français, Européens et Américains face à l'alimentation.* Paris: Odile Jacob, 2008.

Georgia

Population: 4,555,911 (July 2013 est.)

Population Rank: 122nd

Population Growth Rate: −0.33% (2013 est.)

Life Expectancy at Birth: 77.51 years (2013 est.)

Health Expenditures: 9.4% of GDP (2011)

People with Access to Safe Drinking Water: 98% of population (2010 est.)

Average Daily Caloric Consumption: 2,810

Adult Obesity Rate: 22.1% (2008)

Underweight Children under Age 5: 1.1% (2009)

Throughout most of Georgia's history, meat was a luxury, so the Georgians took great advantage of copious fruits, vegetables, and herbs. The bulk of the Georgian culinary repertoire is made up of preparations for vegetables, both cultivated and wild. Over 100 varieties of such wild greens as sarsaparilla, nettles, mallow, ramp, and purslane are still gathered in season and prepared in a surprising number of ways—cooked, marinated, dried for seasoning, or steeped in water for a nutritious drink. But above all, the Georgians enjoy their greens fresh, and no Georgian table is complete without a large platter of leafy cilantro, dill, tarragon, parsley, basil, summer savory, and peppery *tsitsmati,* or falseflax (*Camelina sativa,* similar to arugula). Often there is also *dzhondzholi* (Colchis bladdernut, *Staphylea colchica*), an edible ornamental plant with long stems of tightly furled, beadlike tendrils redolent of garlic. The greens, which are rich in nutrients, provide a refreshing counterpoint to the heavier foods in the meal.

These foods are washed down with wine and local mineral waters like Borzhomi and Nabeghlavi, which have long been touted for their health benefits. To diners used to the mild taste of Perrier or Pellegrino, these waters seem heavy and salty (so much so that Borzhomi is now bottling a Borzhomi Light), but Georgians have traditionally put them to therapeutic use in addition to serving them at the table. Certain foods are also considered especially nutritious. The benefits of yogurt have been touted by Madison Avenue in ads featuring the long-living inhabitants of the Caucasus. Georgians more frequently prescribe *khashi,* a much-loved tripe soup, for digestive problems; it is also a favored hangover remedy when consumed early in the morning following a drinking bout. The marigold petals used in place of saffron are also said to aid in digestion, while *nadugi,* the delicious whey derived from cow milk and often served mixed with fresh herbs, is virtually fat-free and is considered a sclerosis preventative. The traditional Georgian diet is notable for its high amount of omega-3 fats, found in walnuts, walnut oil, and purslane. Purslane contains more omega-3s than any other leafy green vegetable.

The 1991 collapse of the Soviet Union ushered in an era of civil unrest and economic pressure. A new generation of Georgians is working to overcome the problems that still plague the country after so many years of dependence on the larger Soviet economy, which provided a ready market for Georgian produce and prepared foods. Although small-scale farms never died out in Georgia, there was plenty of industrial farming to supply the needs of the Russian market, and activists are now working to reestablish sustainable agricultural practices and revive the legendary wines that had either disappeared from the market or been restyled for the Russian palate. In the twenty-first century Georgia is a small country with a shattered infrastructure, but it is placing a good measure of economic hope on fairly traditional, organic agriculture.

Darra Goldstein

Further Reading

Goldstein, Darra. *The Georgian Feast: The Vibrant Culture and Savory Food of the Republic of Georgia.* Berkeley: University of California Press, 1999.

Holisky, Dee Ann. "The Rules of the *Supra* or How to Drink in Georgian." *Annual of the Society for the Study of Caucasia* 1 (1989): 22–40.

Germany

Population: 81,147,265 (July 2013 est.)
Population Rank: 16th
Population Growth Rate: –0.19% (2013 est.)
Life Expectancy at Birth: 80.32 years (2013 est.)
Health Expenditures: 11.1% of GDP (2011)
People with Access to Safe Drinking Water: 100% of population (2010 est.)
Average Daily Caloric Consumption: 3,530
Adult Obesity Rate: 25.1% (2008)
Underweight Children under Age 5: 1.1% (2006)

For most Germans, diet and health are closely linked. This could be traced back to the holistic approaches to medicine that were practiced in medieval times, and thus to its roots in India, where it is still alive in the Ayurvedic school. But with collective morality loosening, moral obligations have become more individualized and today include the obligation to eat right, that is, healthily.

Life expectancy in Germany is increasing; as of 2013, it is at more than 75 years for men (of which more than 68 years are spent in good health) and more than 81 for women (of which 72 in good health). But it is still thought that nutritional knowledge is insufficient. Overall alcohol consumption is decreasing, and there is a trend toward eating poultry and fish instead of red meat, but fat consumption remains too high and not enough vegetables and fruit are eaten. Varying levels of education, financial means, and gender make for different patterns. The higher social classes and women have significantly better nutritional knowledge than the lower classes and men, respectively.

According to a survey conducted in 2003, 66.9 percent of all German men are overweight, with a body mass index (BMI) of 25 or above, including 17.1 percent who are obese, with a BMI of 30 or above. As in most Western countries, slimness is seen as an ideal and is projected as such in the media. In its most excessive forms, for instance, in fashion advertising, it is also publicly criticized. The link to eating disorders, which are seen as psychological in origin, is widely accepted. Seventy percent of girls between 14 and 15 years are thought to have a diet history. Indeed, diets are an ever-present subject in newspapers, magazines, and books.

Food production, preparation, and trade are strongly regulated in contemporary Germany. The *Lebensmittelrecht* (food law) is a federal law falling under the jurisdiction of both the Ministry for Consumer Protection and the Ministry for Health. Its main purpose is to guarantee food safety as well as a certain level of quality. Looked at rationally and put into a larger perspective, most food scares and scandals seem somewhat overblown when set against the actual casualties. Undoubtedly, objective food safety in Germany has never been as high as today, and the crisis surrounding bovine spongiform encephalopathy (mad cow disease), for instance, became a turning point in German food politics, as from that point transparency and organic agriculture were heavily promoted.

Genetically engineered food is a very controversial topic in Germany, where the first experimental plantings have only recently been allowed.

Another discussion concerns ingredients seen as potential allergens or for those who are subject to lactose, gluten, and other food intolerances.

Insecurity and angst resulting from the inability to understand the often-complex interrelations between diet and health combine with a romanticization of supposedly pure natural food versus artificial human-made food. This has led to a rise in vegetarianism—these days about 8 percent of all Germans are vegetarians—as well as growing environmental awareness, apparent in a multitude of ecological groups, notable among them the Green Party.

But many today apply *gesunder Menschenverstand* (literally, healthy common sense) to seek a balance between human-scale artisanal and industrial perfection in food. Healthy alternatives take different forms for different people. Abstention from smoking, alcohol, and/or sweets during Lent (the weeks leading up to Easter) is not necessarily linked to religious practice. Homeopathic treatment is gradually being recognized by health insurers. Pharmacies expand to become health centers. Ayurvedic treatment is in, and yoga schools are booming. But most important is the growing market for organic and biodynamic food, led by small chains of organic supermarkets. Customers are mainly families with young children from the middle to upper classes, but generally, in spite of discussions about what is acceptable as such, the organic alternative, though not affordable for all, is seen as the better option for reasons beyond personal health.

Ursula Heinzelmann

Further Reading

Anderson, Jean, and Hedy Würz. *The New German Cookbook.* New York: HarperCollins, 1993.

Heinzelmann, Ursula. *Food Culture in Germany.* Westport, CT: Greenwood Press, 2008.

Great Britain

United Kingdom:
Population: 63,395,574 (July 2013 est.)
Population Rank: 22nd
Population Growth Rate: 0.55% (2013 est.)
Life Expectancy at Birth: 80.29 years (2013 est.)
Health Expenditures: 9.3% of GDP (2011)
People with Access to Safe Drinking Water: 100% of population (2010 est.)

Average Daily Caloric Consumption: 3,440
Adult Obesity Rate: 26.9% (2008)
Underweight Children under Age 5: Unknown or negligible

There are variations in diet according to region and income group—the Scots eat especially high levels of salt, sugar, and fat, while people in the southeast of England spend the most on fruit and vegetables. Low-income families tend to resist change and avoid experiments with new foods. Substantial minorities observe special diets, based on religious (kosher, halal, Hindu) or ethical (vegetarian, vegan) requirements.

A lack of food is rare, as are diseases due to dietary deficiencies, although nutritionists express concern over intakes of certain micronutrients, particularly vitamin D and iron in some groups of the population. More problems are related to overnutrition including high intakes of fat, refined carbohydrates, and salt and the associated obesity, cardiovascular disease, diabetes, and hypertension. Levels of obesity (a body mass index of over 30) have increased significantly in the past three to four decades, especially among children and adolescents. Cardiovascular disease is a major cause of premature death in the United Kingdom, and there is evidence for a link to diet, as with the high incidence of type 2 diabetes. High alcohol intake among some groups is also a concern.

The official advice is to reduce the proportion of energy derived from fat and increase that from complex carbohydrates in the diet, and to increase intakes of vegetables and fruit. Encouraging higher consumption of these is an official priority, promoted in various ways, including provision of fruit in primary schools and a campaign called "Eat Five a Day" (five portions of fruit or vegetables).

Consciousness of food hygiene has become increasingly important, as more food is pre-prepared and held in a partially or fully cooked state; intensive farming and industrial processing have also given rise to concerns about pathogens ranging from salmonella in eggs to bovine spongiform encephalopathy (BSE, or mad cow disease) in beef. Responses have ranged from public health measures, such as tightening legislation relating to food safety, to individual choice in pursuit of organically grown food. Most food-borne illnesses are probably related to *E. coli* 0157, salmonella, *Listeria monocytogenes,* campylobacter, and *Clostridium perfringens.* Less quantifiable threats are BSE, pesticide residues, irradiation, and genetic modification, all recurrently the subject of intense debate and suspicion.

Relative perceptions of the risk to health from diet vary between health professionals, the media, and the public. Health professionals consider poor diet and food-borne bacteria or viruses as the highest risks. The media concentrate on "scares" and stories with sensational and sinister implications. The public, nervous about an industrialized food supply and cynical of advertising, tends to choose on the basis of personal likes and dislikes, fashion, and convenience.

Laura Mason

Roast Beef and Yorkshire Pudding

About 5 lb beef sirloin or rib, preferably from a traditional breed fed on grass
Salt, pepper, and a little dry mustard powder mixed with about 1 tbsp flour

For the Pudding
4 oz (1 scant cup) all-purpose flour
Pinch of salt
2 eggs
5 fl oz milk and 5 fl oz water, mixed

Dust the fat of the meat with the flour mixture. Put the joint in a roasting pan and start in a very hot oven (475°F), for about 20 minutes. Turn the temperature down to 375°F, and cook for 15 minutes per pound (rare), plus 15 extra minutes (for medium-rare), plus 30 minutes extra (for well-done). Remove the meat from the oven, and put it on a heated plate in a warm place. Leave to rest for 30 minutes before carving.

While the meat cooks, put the flour for the pudding in a bowl, and add a pinch of salt. Break in the eggs, and stir well. Add the milk and water slowly, stirring well. The batter should be the consistency of light cream. When the meat comes out of the oven, take a roasting pan and add about a tablespoonful of drippings from the meat. Heat it in the oven for a few minutes at 450°F. Remove the pan from the oven, and pour in the batter (wear oven gloves, as the fat may spit). Return to the oven, and bake for 30–40 minutes, until golden and rumpled. Cut into squares for serving.

Make the gravy in the pan the meat was cooked in. Pour all the fat and juices into a small bowl. Spoon off the fat, and reserve the juices. Add about a tablespoon of fat back to the pan, and stir in a tablespoon of flour. Stir over gentle heat until the mixture is lightly browned. Then blend in the juices from cooking the meat and some stock (or water from cooking vegetables or a gravy mix) to make a thin sauce. Cook gently for a few minutes, adjust the seasoning, and serve with the beef and Yorkshire pudding.

Further Reading

Mason, Laura. *Food Culture in Great Britain.* Westport, CT: Greenwood Press, 2004.

Mason, Laura, and Catherine Brown. *Taste of Britain.* London: HarperCollins, 2007.

Oddy, Derek. *From Plain Fare to Fusion Food: British Diet from the 1890s to the 1990s.* Woodbridge, UK: Boydell Press, 2004.

Greece

Population: 10,772,967 (July 2013 est.)
Population Rank: 81st
Population Growth Rate: 0.04% (2013 est.)
Life Expectancy at Birth: 80.18 years (2013 est.)
Health Expenditures: 9% of GDP (2011)
People with Access to Safe Drinking Water: 100% of population (2010 est.)
Average Daily Caloric Consumption: 3,700
Adult Obesity Rate: 20.1% (2008)
Underweight Children under Age 5: Unknown or Negligible

For Greeks, food is basic for the healthy balance of the body and mind. This is obvious in the relationship that Greek cuisine has with natural products. Fresh produce and ingredients are fundamental to Greek cuisine not only for their better taste but also for their nutritional value.

Greek food is highly seasonal and localized. Greeks believe that local products are always best. In addition, the long history of farming and well-established traditions assure its people that the products they get are appropriate for their health. The diet has even been recognized throughout the world as the so-called Mediterranean diet, which is based on fresh local products, eaten in moderation. Modern industrialized farming makes Greek people unsure about the quality and safety of products since, according to their beliefs, when money is involved in such mass production, there is little personal care by the farmers for their products.

Greeks believe that healthy food means cooked food and that the longer it cooks, the better it is. It is only recently that Greek people might enjoy a medium-cooked steak, and even now it is highly unlikely to find this as a home-cooked meal. For Greeks, the application of fire kills any type of bacteria or germs that might exist on vegetables.

In addition, religion is highly connected with diet and health in Greece. In the Greek Orthodox Church there are several long periods of fasting (*Sarakosti*). There is a period before Christmas for about 30 days; the *megali sarakosti* (Lent) before Easter, which lasts for a bit longer than 40 days; and finally the 15-day sarakosti before August 15, when the Virgin Mary is celebrated. Although many people do not actually believe in these long periods of abstinence from animal products, they do follow it since they believe that it is very good for the body and cleans out all the toxins. At the same time, the church has carefully devised the diet so people get all the necessary nutrients.

A healthy diet and the use of natural products are also important for medical purposes. Greeks are generally aware of the nutritious properties of foods. For example, they know that tomatoes, lentils, and beets contain a lot of iron. Thus they try to combine or use ingredients so as to include all the important nutrients in their diet. However, certain combinations are used for various more serious health issues. Greek coffee dissolved in lemon is highly recommended for diarrhea. *Glistrida* (purslane) is considered to be medicine for high cholesterol, onions for people with high blood pressure, garlic for those with low blood pressure, and so on.

Evidently, although Greece is a modern, Westernized, progressive country, people have a special bond with food and as a consequence with nature. They follow the seasonal life cycles with the celebration of different occasions, and they understand food as the transformation of nature into something tasty that fulfills, follows, and emphasizes important phases of life.

Giorgos Maltezakis

Further Reading

Dalby, Andrew. *Food in the Ancient World from A to Z.* Oxford: Routledge, 2003.

Sterling, Richard, Kate Reeves, and Georgia Dacakis. *World Food Greece: For People Who Live to Eat, Drink, and Travel.* Oakland, CA: Lonely Planet, 2002.

Gypsies

The many impoverished Gypsies of eastern Europe and the camps of western Europe have poor health due to inadequate and unbalanced diets as well as generally poor living conditions and poor health care. But even middle-class

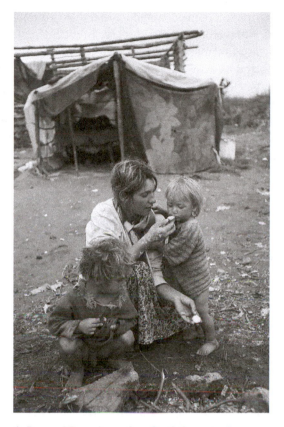

A Roma (Gypsy) mother feeds her son in a temporary home in a poor settlement in Romania. Many Roma have little access to electricity or healthy foods. (Sean Gallup/Getty Images)

and wealthier Gypsies often have health problems resulting from unhealthy diets and lifestyles. Studies of American Roma have demonstrated that the diet, which is high in salt, sugar, and animal fat, together with a lack of aerobic exercise and a nearly universal prevalence of smoking, leads to very high levels of blood cholesterol, triglycerides, and blood sugar. Abnormally high blood pressure usually begins before 30 years of age. By age 50, nearly 100 percent are afflicted with diabetes and vascular disease. Roma generally are considered old if over 55. Heart attacks occur in the early 30s, even the late 20s. Some Romani families eat only fish and vegetables for Lent, but there is a general opinion in the community that this Lenten diet is unhealthy, even for patients with cardiovascular disease. In recent years there has been some improvement as many members of the community have become more health conscious and as smoking has somewhat decreased, but as yet there are no recent studies to confirm this.

Dietary problems have been compounded historically by a cultural bias for obesity. To be fat was to be powerful; thinness was a sign of weakness. The term in Romani for a traditional leader is *Rom Baro,* or "big man." While meant in the sense of political power, it is also almost always literally true.

William G. Lockwood

Further Reading

Edwards, D. M., and R. G. Watt. "Diet and Hygiene in the Life of Gypsy Travelers in Hertfordshire." *Community and Dental Health* 14 (1997): 41–46.

Leo, Jacey. *Gypsy Open-Fire Cookbook.* Baltimore, MD: PublishAmerica, 2005.

Hungary

Population: 9,939,470 (July 2013 est.)
Population Rank: 87th
Population Growth Rate: –0.2% (2013 est.)
Life Expectancy at Birth: 75.24 years (2013 est.)
Health Expenditures: 7.7% of GDP (2011)
People with Access to Safe Drinking Water: 100% of population (2010 est.)
Average Daily Caloric Consumption: 3,440
Adult Obesity Rate: 27.6% (2008)
Underweight Children under Age 5: Unknown or Negligible

Like much of central and eastern Europe, Hungary is struggling with the long-term effects of its traditional diet, as well as of the Communist-era agricultural policies and lifestyles that resulted in meat-centric and fat-heavy diets. Obesity is the number-one public health problem in Hungary, according to studies, with some estimates putting the number of obese adults at more than 15 percent of the population.

Both age and location greatly affect the way that Hungarians cook and eat. Hungarians living in rural areas tend to eat in the most traditional manner and, ironically, often have less access to a variety of fresh fruit and vegetables, as well as the many organic food shops that stock whole grains, than Budapest residents do. Although sunflower oil is increasingly being used, pork fat remains heavily used by many older people who do not take advantage of healthier options now available.

Age is also an important factor in determining lifestyle and health. While the older generation is fairly set in its ways in terms of cooking and eating, younger Hungarians, particularly those living in urban areas, are more likely to cook non-Hungarian and lower-fat recipes. They tend to avoid the abundance of deep-fried dishes and sugary sweets, and they like to shop at organic shops and markets when they can afford to.

In addition to the diet, since the fall of Communism, experts have noted that lifestyles have become less active—in part due to the easier access to cars and the arrival of multiple television channels—with people walking less and not exercising enough. Alcoholism, too, is a serious health problem in Hungary, with mortality due to alcoholism three times higher than the European Union average for males and 2.5 times higher for females.

Carolyn Bánfalvi

Gulyás (Goulash)

Goulash is an everyday dish served at nearly every Hungarian restaurant. It is so simple to make that any Hungarian who cooks can do it. Many also cook it over an open fire in a bogrács (cauldron), which adds a smoky flavor. Some cooks add pinched pasta (csipetke) before serving. If you were to continue cooking the meat without adding water or potatoes, the resulting dish would be pörkölt, which is the stew that foreigners tend to think of as goulash. Gulyás is an everyday meal, eaten with thick-crusted white bread.

4 tbsp sunflower or canola oil
2 yellow onions, chopped
1 1/2 lb beef chuck, trimmed and cut into 1/2-in. cubes
Kosher salt and freshly ground black pepper, to taste
1/4 c sweet paprika
2 tsp dried marjoram
2 tsp caraway seeds
2 cloves garlic, finely chopped
2 medium carrots, cut into 1/2-in. cubes
2 medium parsnips, cut into 1/2-in. cubes
1 1/2 lb medium-sized new potatoes, peeled and cut into 1/2-in. cubes

1 tomato, cored and chopped
1 Italian frying pepper, chopped

Heat the oil in a pot over medium heat. Add the onions, cover, and cook, stirring occasionally, until soft and translucent, about 10 minutes. Increase the heat to high. Add the beef, and season with salt and pepper. Cook, uncovered, until the meat is lightly browned, about 6 minutes. Stir in the paprika, marjoram, caraway, and garlic, and cook until fragrant, about 2 minutes. Add the carrots, parsnips, and 5 cups water. Bring to a boil; reduce heat to medium. Simmer, covered, until the beef is nearly tender, about 40 minutes. Add the potatoes, and cook, uncovered, until tender, about 25 minutes. Stir in the tomatoes and pepper; cook for 2 minutes. Season with salt and pepper to taste.

Further Reading

Bánfalvi, Carolyn. *Food Wine Budapest.* New York: Little Bookroom, 2008.

Koerner, Andras. *A Taste of the Past: The Daily Life and Cooking of a Nineteenth-Century Hungarian Jewish Homemaker.* Durham, NH: University Press of New England, 2003.

Iceland

Population: 315,281 (July 2013 est.)
Population Rank: 179th
Population Growth Rate: 0.66% (2013 est.)
Life Expectancy at Birth: 81.11 years (2013 est.)
Health Expenditures: 9.1% of GDP (2011)
People with Access to Safe Drinking Water: 100% of population (2010 est.)
Average Daily Caloric Consumption: 3,330
Adult Obesity Rate: 23.2% (2008)
Underweight Children under Age 5: Unknown or Negligible

There is no better indication that the Icelandic diet has been lauded and commended for its organic, hormone-free nature than the fact that many countries are importing its meats and fish—in fact, with Whole Foods Market in the United States heavily marketing its selection of Icelandic lamb and skýr, these mainstays of the country's diet have indeed entered mainstream popular culture.

The strong reliance on fish, pasture-raised lamb, and wild game for food means the Icelandic diet is rich in omega-3 fats; some experts attribute the low depression rates, despite the bleak climate, to this.

By consuming geothermally grown vegetables, wild berries, and whole grains such as barley and rye, Icelanders absorb a lot of antioxidants, which keep them healthy during the icy months.

Desiree Koh

Further Reading

Rognvaldardottir, Nanna. *Cool Cuisine: Traditional Icelandic Cuisine*. Reykjavík, Iceland: Vaka-Helgafell, 2004.

Wilcox, Jonathan, and Zawiah Abdul Latif. *Iceland*. New York: Marshall Cavendish Benchmark, 2007.

Ireland

Population: 4,775,982 (July 2013 est.)
Population Rank: 119th
Population Growth Rate: 1.16% (2013 est.)
Life Expectancy at Birth: 80.44 years (2013 est.)
Health Expenditures: 9.4% of GDP (2011)
People with Access to Safe Drinking Water: 100% of population (2010 est.)
Average Daily Caloric Consumption: 3,530
Adult Obesity Rate: 25.2% (2008)
Underweight Children under Age 5: Unknown or Negligible

Cardiovascular disease is the main cause of death in Ireland, accounting for 36 percent of all deaths and including heart attacks, strokes, and other circulatory diseases. The government has been working with the food industry to reduce salt levels in processed food and is involved in promoting a more active lifestyle among the population. Research shows that certain segments of the community are more likely to suffer from diet-related illnesses. In a study, the contribution of fat to total energy intake increased as socioeconomic status decreased, a finding reflective of the higher consumption of foods high in fat by respondents from socially disadvantaged groups. Energy from carbohydrates was greatest among those from socially advantaged groups and was close to the recommended 50 percent of the total energy intake. Conversely, energy from protein decreased with increasing social status in groups. The mean intake of vitamins and minerals was generally close to or above the recommended values. Another diet-related health issue in Ireland is the amount of alcohol consumed, which is significantly higher than the European average.

Máirtín Mac Con Iomaire

Further Reading

Andrews, Colman. *The Country Cooking of Ireland.* San Francisco: Chronicle Books, 2009.

Clarkson, Louis A., and E. Margaret Crawford. *Feast and Famine, Food and Nutrition in Ireland 1500–1900.* Oxford: Oxford University Press, 2001.

Italy

Population: 61,482,297 (July 2013 est.)
Population Rank: 23rd
Population Growth Rate: 0.34% (2013 est.)
Life Expectancy at Birth: 81.95 years (2013 est.)
Health Expenditures: 9.5% of GDP (2011)
People with Access to Safe Drinking Water: 100% of population (2010 est.)
Average Daily Caloric Consumption: 3,660
Adult Obesity Rate: 19.8% (2008)
Underweight Children under Age 5: Unknown or Negligible

Since the late 1950s, there have been radical changes in the amount and the composition of the foods that Italians consume. For centuries, populations around the Mediterranean Sea, including Italians, had to strive against food scarcity, tilling soils that were often less than generous and making do with what they could grow around them. As a consequence, the diet was based mostly on carbohydrates, pulses, and vegetables, with little fat and animal protein.

Then, starting from the end of World War II, even the less-well-off became able to afford a more diverse and abundant diet. Nutrition patterns changed under the influence of new packaging and conservation techniques, industrial mass production, and more sophisticated systems of distribution. A widespread economic development that led to the actual boom in the 1960s allowed many to lead better lives and enjoy a more regular intake of food, even though it often severed the ties to their traditional ways of life, including culinary habits. The daily energy intake passed from slightly below 2,000 calories in the 1950s to almost 3,500 nowadays. Italians are consuming more meat and sugar, and coronary diseases are reaping more victims than ever before, because of fattier and higher-calorie diets. Obesity, especially in children, has become a main concern for the Ministry of Health, which has launched public campaigns aiming to educate the parents and the children themselves to eat better.

At the same time, the whole world seems to have discovered that the way the Mediterranean people had eaten for centuries in their effort to fight hunger actually constitutes a very healthy diet. The international public became aware of the advantages of the so-called Mediterranean diet in the late 1980s, when scientist Ancel Keys and a group of researchers published the results of the survey they had conducted in seven countries. Then, in 1990, the U.S. Department of Agriculture issued dietary guidelines for Americans that become the basis for the 1992 Food Guide Pyramid, clearly shaped by Keys's findings in southern Italy back in the 1950s. However, because of the way the media describe it, it is unclear whether the Mediterranean diet is considered as a cultural and historical construction, as a selection of specific foods, or, more scientifically, as a nutrient profile.

Despite the changes in their dietary patterns, and the regional differences, Italians still tend to eat more carbohydrates, legumes, and vegetables than Americans do. The distribution within these categories has changed, too: from the 1950s, the growing availability of bread and pasta marked a decrease in the consumption of other cereals considered less desirable, such as barley or rye. Rice and maize maintained a certain acceptance in northern regions. The southern regions traditionally consume larger quantities of carbohydrates and vegetables than the northern ones. With regard to the consumption of different kinds of meat, beef increased until the 1970s, reaching a constant level that suddenly decreased at the end of the 1990s, due to the mad cow scare and other health-related anxieties. In contrast, consumption of chicken, pork, and rabbit is growing, on account of the lower prices of these meats and the fact that Italians now consider them as nutritious as beef.

Dietary rules change during each individual's lifetime. A very special moment for many women is pregnancy. Gaining weight in the months preceding the birth of a baby is not only considered acceptable but even recommended. Most women opt for breast-feeding, considered better for the child, since it creates a closer connection with the mother and provides the child with all necessary nutrients and a better protection against infections and diseases. For this reason, breast-feeding in public is socially accepted.

Up to 5 months of age, babies are fed exclusively milk or formula. From 5 to 12 months, babies are weaned, and new flavors and foods are introduced into their diet. Between one and three years of age, the babies are supposed to adapt their diet to the adults' habits. The goal is to let babies get used to the taste of real food, since there is no concept of baby food per se. At this point, babies are usually more than happy to start eating what their parents and other adults eat, especially at social occasions when many people are gathered around the table. There are no children's menus in restaurants: children are supposed to eat small portions of the same dishes the adults are having. Children are often curious to taste adult food, and in many families it is accepted to serve them even tiny drops of coffee in their milk and also wine, often diluted in lots of water.

There is no concept of food for the old. Senior citizens are supposed to eat the way they always did, unless they have specific ailments or suffer from loss of teeth. They continue to drink wine with their meals, to have their coffee in the morning, to season their dishes with salt, and to consume fried food and sweets. Since the calorie intake does not decrease, while retirement implies a less active style of life, it is quite common for older people to gain weight and to suffer from problems connected with high levels of cholesterol in the blood, high blood pressure, and diabetes.

Most physicians in Italy are not particularly interested in matters of nutrition, unless they affect some specific ailments. With the exception of pediatricians, who are definitely more involved in the subject, and also because of pressure from mothers, many physicians do not even take that subject during their professional training. For this reason, the advice some medical doctors give is quite vague, often based more on common sense than on study and research. Most of the knowledge people get about their food and their nutritional needs comes from less reliable sources: the media. Most television channels, newspapers, and magazines have a section on health, which often deals with food-related issues.

Fabio Parasecoli

Further Reading

Dickie, John. *Delizia! The Epic History of the Italians and Their Food.* New York: Free Press, 2008.

Heltosky, Carol. *Garlic and Oil: Food and Politics in Italy.* Oxford: Berg, 2006.

Montanari, Massimo, and Alberto Capatti. *Italian Cuisine: A Cultural History.* New York: Columbia University Press, 2003.

Parasecoli, Fabio. *Food Culture in Italy.* Westport, CT: Greenwood Press, 2004.

Latvia

Population: 2,178,443 (July 2013 est.)
Population Rank: 143rd
Population Growth Rate: −0.61% (2013 est.)
Life Expectancy at Birth: 73.19 years (2013 est.)
Health Expenditures: 6.7% of GDP (2010)
People with Access to Safe Drinking Water: 99% of population (2010 est.)
Average Daily Caloric Consumption: 3,020
Adult Obesity Rate: 24.9% (2008)
Underweight Children under Age 5: Unknown or Negligible

In combination with a high-fat diet, modernization has led to a decrease in exercise in Latvia and therefore an increased threat of cholesterol-related health issues. Alcohol consumption is high and is one of the main causes of traffic deaths, fires, and crime. Smoking is also common, and illnesses such as emphysema, lung cancer, and asthma continue to present problems.

Neil L. Coletta

Skaba Putra (Sour Barley Porridge)

1/4 c finely ground cracked barley
1/2 tsp salt
2 c buttermilk
2 c milk (whole or skim)
1/3 c sour cream
Pork fat (or bacon), sautéed (optional)
Onions, sautéed (optional)

In a large pot, mix barley and salt with 1 cup water, and slowly bring to a boil. Reduce heat to low, cover, and simmer for 45 minutes, or until barley is tender and water has been absorbed. Set aside to cool slightly.

Add buttermilk and milk, and stir to the consistency of a thick soup. Cover and store overnight (or up to 12 hours) in a warm place so that the porridge sours slightly. Refrigerate for at least one full day to continue the fermentation, which will intensify over time.

Add sour cream before serving, as well as the optional pork fat (or bacon) and onions.

Further Reading

O'Connor, Kevin. *Culture and Customs of the Baltic States.* Westport, CT: Greenwood Press, 2006.

Pigozne-Brinkmane, Ieva. *The Cuisine of Latvia.* Rīga: Latvian Institute, 2004.

Lithuania

Population: 3,515,858 (July 2013 est.)
Population Rank: 132nd
Population Growth Rate: –0.28% (2013 est.)
Life Expectancy at Birth: 75.77 years (2013 est.)
Health Expenditures: 7% of GDP (2010)
People with Access to Safe Drinking Water: 92% of population (2000 est.)
Average Daily Caloric Consumption: 3,420
Adult Obesity Rate: 27.6% (2008)
Underweight Children under Age 5: Unknown or Negligible

In response to the changing perceptions about healthy diets, since the early 1990s there has been a major change in local cooking methods, moving away from animal fat to vegetable oils. Even in the early 1990s, most of the food was still cooked either in pig fat or, on rare occasions, in butter. Rapeseed oil (canola) was used for frying fish. Today, extra-virgin and virgin olive oil and other vegetable oils have made inroads into everyday diets, and pig fat has disappeared from the supermarket shelves. While there is a widespread perception that fat is not good for one's health, health-conscious eating is mostly practiced by the younger generations, who did not experience the food scarcity in the early Socialist era. As in other places around the world, dieting is usually practiced among young women, who tend to ration their daily caloric intakes following dietary fashions. There is also an increased interest in traditional medicine, especially the use of local herbs' medicinal powers for healing. While such knowledge survived in Lithuania during the early decades of the twentieth century, which brought the industrialization and professionalization of medicine, and continued to be practiced in most homes under Socialism, today it is receiving a renewed interest.

Diana Mincyte

Further Reading

Bindokienė, Danutė Brazytė. *Papročiai ir Tradicijos Išeivijoje/Lithuanian Customs and Traditions.* 1989. Chicago: Lithuanian World Community, 1998.

Imbrasienė, Birutė, ed. *Lithuanian Traditional Foods.* Vilnius, Lithuania: Baltos Lankos, 1998.

Malta

Population: 411,277 (July 2013 est.)
Population Rank: 175th
Population Growth Rate: 0.34% (2013 est.)
Life Expectancy at Birth: 79.98 years (2013 est.)
Health Expenditures: 8.5% of GDP (2010)
People with Access to Safe Drinking Water: 100% of population (2010 est.)
Average Daily Caloric Consumption: 3,590
Adult Obesity Rate: 28.8% (2008)
Underweight Children under Age 5: Unknown or Negligible

Since the latter half of the twentieth century, Malta has witnessed a shift toward Westernized dietary patterns, with an increased consumption of meat, dairy products, and processed high-fat, high-sugar, high-salt foods and a

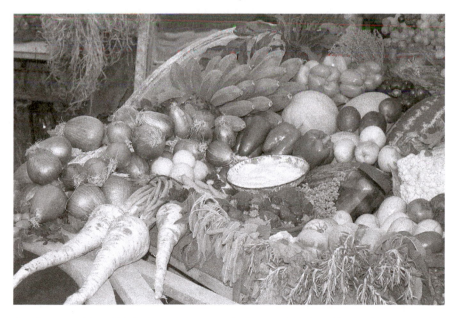

A selection of local Maltese produce on display in a farming village. (Shutterstock)

decreased consumption of pulses. Common foods in children's diets are chicken nuggets, burgers, pizzas, and packet noodles, together with a variety of packaged salted snacks, chocolate or jam-filled croissants, and cookies.

In 1988, the "National Nutrient Goals and Dietary Guidelines" document specifically recommended that Maltese eat less meat and consume fish and poultry in preference to beef; replace high-fat dairy products with low-fat alternatives; and eat fewer eggs and more fresh fruit and vegetables and whole-grain cereal products.

Following a traditional Maltese diet would go some way toward meeting these recommendations. For example, rabbit is one of the meats lowest in fat, whereas fish is used in several recipes ranging from *aljotta* (a broth-type fish soup containing rice and some vegetables), to pulpetti, to torta tal-lampuki. Moreover, fresh seasonal vegetables are used, raw or boiled and then cooled, to make vegetable salads, as well as a variety of soups. *Tadam mimli* (stuffed tomatoes), *brunġiel mimli* (stuffed eggplants), and *bżar mimli* (stuffed bell peppers) are three common traditional dishes in which the vegetables are filled either with rice and meat or with rice, tuna, olives, and capers and then baked.

Fruit, which is lauded for its health benefits, is luckily a staple in the diet. Different local fruits are available year-round, including plums, peaches, nectarines, apricots, pears, oranges, tangerines, strawberries, melons, watermelons, and grapes. Some claim that one of the best local fruits is prickly pears, which grow on the side of country lanes. Cut first thing in the morning and peeled after they have been soaked in water to tame the spines, prickly pears are delicious eaten cold from the refrigerator. They come in shades of red, green, and orange and are a feast for the eye when presented on the table in a bowl.

Local grapes are also pressed to make a variety of wines, and the elders insist that a glass of wine daily proffers many health benefits. Interestingly, some local entrepreneurs are using prickly pears, pomegranates, and various herbs to make liquors that all have a distinctive Mediterranean aroma and are marketed with an emphasis on their natural ingredients.

Suzanne Piscopo

Further Reading

Billiard, E. "When Tradition Becomes Trendy: Social Distinction in Maltese Food." *Anthropological Notebooks* 12 (2006): 113–26.

Caruana, Claudia. *Taste of Malta.* New York: Hippocrene, 1998.

Caruana Galizia, Anne, and Helen Caruana Galizia. *The Food and Cookery of Malta.* London: Pax Books, 1999.

Moldova

Population: 3,619,925 (July 2013 est.)
Population Rank: 130th
Population Growth Rate: −1.02% (2013 est.)
Life Expectancy at Birth: 69.82 years (2013 est.)
Health Expenditures: 11.4% of GDP (2011)
People with Access to Safe Drinking Water: 96% of population (2010 est.)
Average Daily Caloric Consumption: 2,910
Adult Obesity Rate: 21.2% (2008)
Underweight Children under Age 5: 3.2% (2005)

Like many other ex-Soviet states, the population of Moldova does not score as well as most western Europeans in many key health indicators. Also, like many other countries dealing with post-Soviet stresses, many of the health issues are related to lifestyle, including smoking, alcohol consumption, and diet. Food shortages are, and have been, a reality for many people and often result in inadequate nutritional intake. An example of this occurred during the recent 2007 drought, which drastically reduced food reserves. This in turn led to a national health problem because the Moldovan population relies heavily on the food it produces.

Even though Moldova produces a large amount of fruit and vegetables and these also feature heavily in the cuisine, at times consumption has been low and nutrient intake poor due to poverty and poor yields. In the time of large collective farms, Moldova had a high use of pesticides and herbicides. There may be environmental remnants from this time, but today produce is often cleaner and more organic, since Moldova now has a low use of pesticides and fertilizers. For many households, the fruit and vegetables that they grow or buy are likely to be of high quality.

Kate Johnston

Further Reading

Agriculture and Agro-Food Industry of the Republic of Moldova. Chisinau, Moldova: Ministry of Agriculture and Food Industry, 2009

Buzila, Varvara, and Teodorina Bazgu. "Ritual Breads through the Season." In *Culinary Cultures of Europe: Identity, Diversity and Dialogue,* edited by Darra Goldstein and Kathrin Merkle. Strasbourg, France: Council of Europe Publishing, 2005.

The Netherlands

Population: 16,805,037 (July 2013 est.)
Population Rank: 64th
Population Growth Rate: 0.44% (2013 est.)
Life Expectancy at Birth: 81.01 years (2013 est.)
Health Expenditures: 12% of GDP (2011)
People with Access to Safe Drinking Water: 100% of population (2010 est.)
Average Daily Caloric Consumption: 3,240
Adult Obesity Rate: 18.8% (2008)
Underweight Children under Age 5: Unknown or Negligible

In the Netherlands, traditionally, nutritional value is considered more important than gastronomic pleasure and the palatability of food. Before and after World War II, many middle-class women were educated in domestic science at schools. Apart from home economics and hygiene, these schools taught and advocated a frugal diet with a high nutritional value. The schools published highly popular cookbooks that greatly influenced domestic cooking and future generations of domestic cooks.

At the same time, so as to prevent chronic diseases, the Dutch government's food policy started strongly focusing on health and food-safety issues. Due to food shortages during World War II and the need to feed the nation, historically the Dutch government and governmental organizations are well enmeshed with the local food industries and factories. Nowadays, a healthy diet is often advocated via media campaigns that promote the consumption of national agricultural produce and industrial products.

During the postwar era, Het Voedingscentrum (the Nutrition Center) became the most important and best-known governmental organization for nutritional information for citizens. Connecting scientific insights with a healthy diet and the daily practice of consumers, in the 1950s it successfully developed a food classification system that informs the general population on how to eat healthy and safely. Nutrition information is provided through *De Schijf van Vijf* (the five disks), via which the so-called whole food assortment is divided. It is comparable to the U.S. Food Pyramid. Depending on the group, the focus is on the amount of dietary fiber, saturated fat, energy, and/or specific micronutrients contained in the food products.

In comparison to other European countries, there are considerable differences in dietary patterns and consumption. Although during the postwar period the availability of foods and food consumption were subject to drastic changes, the Dutch diet remains relatively high in potatoes but also in animal-derived, processed, sweetened, and refined foods. The consumption of vegetables and fruit is similar to the rest of Europe.

The average Dutch citizen is living a longer and a healthier life than in the past. Like elsewhere in the Western world, consumers are tempted by a huge variety of foods available in a growing number of places and in advertising. Subsequently, the pleasures and palatability of food are becoming more important, but today the risks of chronic diseases such as cancer, diabetes, and obesity, and campaigns that focus on health and food safety, remain dominant issues in the minds of Dutch consumers and food policy makers.

Karin Vaneker

Further Reading

Henne Koene, Ada. *Food Shoppers' Guide to Holland.* 4th ed. Delft, the Netherlands: Eburon, 2003.

Rose, Peter R. "The Low Countries." *Encyclopedia of Food and Culture,* edited by Solomon H. Katz, 389–96. New York: Charles Scribner's Sons, 2003.

Norway

Population: 4,722,701 (July 2013 est.)
Population Rank: 120th
Population Growth Rate: 0.33% (2013 est.)
Life Expectancy at Birth: 80.44 years (2013 est.)
Health Expenditures: 9.1% of GDP (2011)
People with Access to Safe Drinking Water: 100% of population (2010 est.)
Average Daily Caloric Consumption: 3,460
Adult Obesity Rate: 21.5% (2008)
Underweight Children under Age 5: Unknown or Negligible

Norwegians are increasingly aware of how important a healthy diet is to prevent serious diseases, for instance, cardiovascular diseases and cancer, which account for the majority of deaths for both men and women. Public campaigns encouraging reductions in the intake of fatty foods and recommending a more substantial consumption of vegetables have made some progress. In general, the diet has improved since 1990, but Norwegians still eat too little greens, fish, and whole-grain bread and too much fat and sugar.

Health authorities recognized the basic problems in diet and nutrition early on. They have made efforts to influence food consumption and eating patterns in accordance with the scientifically elaborated norms for a healthy diet. Norway was one of the first in the world to have an official nutrition policy, established in 1975.

Today, the rapid growth in the food-processing industry has led to an increased demand for legal measures to guarantee certain nutritional standards. The technological development within food production has created new processes and made new additives necessary. One consequence is problems with hygiene and the presence of certain toxic bacteria, for instance, salmonella.

Since 1960, health authorities have worked systematically to reduce the intake of fat and, more particularly, to reduce the percentage of fat in the total energy intake. According to the official recommendations a maximum of 30 percent of the total energy intake should come from fat. There has, in fact, been a real reduction in fat intake since the mid-1980s, from about 40 percent down to about 35 percent, or a little less. Since 2000, there seems to have been no further reduction. This means there is still a long way to go before the ideal goal of 30 percent is reached.

The most important sources of fat in the food consumed by Norwegians are milk and milk products, meat and meat products, and various sorts of household fats, margarine in particular. There has been an increase in the consumption of meat over the last decades, but at the same time, there has been a reduction in the consumption of margarine and in the use of lard and tallow in cooking. The fat intake from milk products has been relatively stable. Fats from milk and butter play a far less important part than before, but the consumption of cream and cheese is up.

According to the Nordic Nutrition Recommendations, people should not get more than 10 percent of their total energy from sugar. The actual percentage has decreased in recent years but is still as high as 14 percent, partly a result of an extraordinarily strong increase in the consumption of sweet carbonated drinks, fruit juices, and confections.

There is clear evidence today supporting the hypothesis that consumption of fruits and vegetables has a protective effect against diseases such as cancer, coronary heart disease, stroke, and diabetes. Fruits and vegetables have a high content of vitamins, minerals, antioxidants, and dietary fiber. A doubling of the consumption of vegetables is assumed to reduce the risk of cancer and cardiovascular diseases substantially. Increased intake of fruits and vegetables may also have an extra effect in replacing less favorable foods in the dietary pattern.

Between 1999 and 2007 there was an increase in the yearly per capita consumption of fruits from 152 to 189 pounds (69 to 86 kilograms) and of vegetables from 132 to 141 pounds (60 to 64 kilograms). However, Norwegians still are not eating enough vegetables, particularly as the highest increase was for tomatoes and cucumbers, that is, vegetables with a high water content. Authorities recommend more fiber-rich vegetables and deeper-colored vegetables. The increase in fruit consumption is primarily due to an increase in the intake of fruit juices.

The consumption differs within populations. Women eat more vegetables, fruits, and berries than men. The consumption is higher in the old-age groups than in the young. Men and women with a higher education eat more fruits and vegetables than people with less education. This has to be taken seriously both in the way educational campaigns are run and also politically in price policies. The increase in the price of fruits and vegetables is high enough to discourage certain low-income groups.

The consumption of potatoes has declined during the last decades. But the health authorities are not so much concerned with the total amount of potato consumption as with the way potatoes are consumed. Today, an increasing amount of potatoes are sold as French fries, chips, and other processed potato products. In Norway only half of the potato consumption is of fresh potatoes. The processed products have high amounts of unhealthy saturated fat.

Campaigns for increased consumption of fish have been going on for several decades. There is clear evidence that high consumption of fish has beneficial effects on health. The main reason is the content in fish of omega-3 fatty acids, even if the contents of iodine, selenine, and vitamin D are also considered important. Omega-3 fatty acids from fish reduce the risk of fatal coronary disease (sudden cardiac death).

Fish is the main dish about seven times a month in Norway, but only 21 percent of the population eats fish three times a week. The consumption of fish is lower than that of meat and far below the recommended quantity. The value of the high consumption is also to some extent reduced because fish is often eaten with saturated fats (margarine, butter).

Experts recommend an increase in the intake of carbohydrates, primarily from whole-grain foods. In addition to vitamins and minerals whole-grain cereals provide natural dietary fiber. A high consumption of such cereals seems to have a beneficial role in reducing the risk of coronary heart disease and a protective effect against the development of hypertension and diabetes. Cereals are the most important source for dietary fiber. Even if more than half of the intake of cereals consists of whole-grain products, the intake is below the recommendations from health authorities.

There is a very high awareness in Norway of the importance of adequate intake of vitamins and minerals, and in some foodstuffs vitamins and minerals are added, to make sure the population gets the necessary amount. In general, a varied diet will cover the necessary intake, and the increased consumption of fruits and vegetables has helped in recent years. But the reduced consumption of fish and increased sugar intake work in the opposite direction.

Most Scandinavians eat too much salt, about 10 grams a day. Too much salt increases the blood pressure and may be a contributing factor to heart disease and stroke. Whereas consumption of meat and fat partly is dependent on individual choice, this is not the case with consumption of salt. How much salt is added during cooking or at the table is not so important, when 75 percent of the salt intake comes from industrially produced foods. This means that the higher the consumption of convenience foods, the higher the intake of salt, and to reduce salt involves far more drastic changes in the food habits.

Henry Notaker

Palesuppe (Bergen Young Saithe Soup)

Many Bergen citizens will insist that the stock has to be made from the entire fish, not only the trimmings, and that a little veal stock should be added to round out the flavor. Some insist that the vegetables have to be cooked separately, and some that the soup is not complete without small fish balls. There are many ways to make a Bergen fish soup, but one common denominator is the rømme, the sour cream.

If saithe is not available, other fishes of the cod family may be used. Instead of or in addition to celeriac, parsnip or leeks may be used.

3 lb young saithe (pollack)
3 pt water
1 tsp salt
2 medium-sized carrots
1 parsley root
1 knob celeriac (celery root)
1/3 c flour
1 1/3 c milk
1/2 c rømme (sour cream)
Chives

Clean and wash the fish, and remove the gills and the eyes. Cut the head in two, and put it in a pot with the tail. Pour in cold water and salt, and bring to a boil. Cut the rest of the fish in slices an inch thick, add to the pot, and let them simmer for a few minutes, then put them aside. Strain the stock. Cut the vegetables into $1/2$-inch dice, and let them boil 5 minutes in the stock. Whisk flour smooth in cold milk, and beat it into the boiling stock. Let it simmer for 5 minutes. Whisk in the sour cream, and sprinkle finely chopped chives over the soup, if desired. Serve the soup first, then the fish with boiled potatoes.

Further Reading

Kjærnes, Unni, ed. *Eating Patterns: A Day in the Lives of Nordic Peoples.* Lysaker, Norway: Lysaker National Institute for Consumer Research, 2001.

Notaker, Henry. *Food Culture in Scandinavia.* Westport, CT: Greenwood Press, 2008.

Viestad, Andreas: *Kitchen of Light: New Scandinavian Cooking.* New York: Artisan, 2003.

Poland

Population: 38,383,809 (July 2013 est.)
Population Rank: 33rd
Population Growth Rate: –0.09% (2013 est.)
Life Expectancy at Birth: 76.45 years (2013 est.)
Health Expenditures: 6.7% of GDP (2011)
People with Access to Safe Drinking Water: 100% of population (2008 est.)
Average Daily Caloric Consumption: 3,400
Adult Obesity Rate: 25.3% (2008)
Underweight Children under Age 5: Unknown or Negligible

Traditional Polish food is rich and heavy. Foods are thickened, flavored, and garnished with dairy, especially sour cream. Meats, including fatty sausages, are daily staples of the national diet. And hardly a dinner is served and eaten without potatoes, pierogi, or both. Time was that most people worked hard to produce the food they ate, and they needed the fat, calories, and protein these foods afforded to survive.

However, modern Poles are not unlike people in the rest of the Western world. They no longer toil each day in the fields. Most Poles are now office

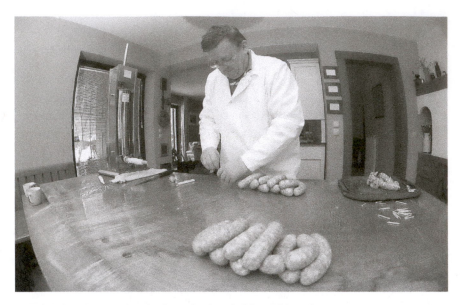

A Polish butcher makes kielbasa by hand. (iStockPhoto)

and factory workers and do not need the high fat and calories of their culture's traditional diet. Also, most Poles are as concerned with fitness as they are with health; they value thin waistlines more than hearty meals. So Poles now eat much less meat than they once did, and their consumption of sour cream and dairy is also down.

Interestingly, though, many elements of traditional Polish cuisine are quite compatible with a modern, healthy diet. For example, in the middle of the last century, the kasha that had long been a staple in Polish diets started to fall out of favor as an old-fashioned, peasant food. Recently, it has experienced a resurgence in popularity due to the increased concern Poles have about dietary fiber and health. Similarly, the traditional cooking oil made with the rapeseed grown on Polish farms is high in the unsaturated fats favored for keeping unhealthy cholesterol levels down. Also, Polish yogurt called kefir has been rediscovered and is gaining popularity among health-conscious Poles.

R. J. Krajewski

Further Reading

Peterson, Joan, and Michael Peterson. *Eat Smart in Poland: How to Decipher the Menu, Know the Market Foods, and Embark on a Tasting Adventure.* Madison, WI: Gingko Press, 2000.

West, Karen. *The Best of Polish Cooking.* New York: Hippocrene Books, 2000.

Portugal

Population: 10,799,270 (July 2013 est.)
Population Rank: 80th
Population Growth Rate: 0.15% (2013 est.)
Life Expectancy at Birth: 78.85 years (2013 est.)
Health Expenditures: 10.4% of GDP (2011)
People with Access to Safe Drinking Water: 99% of population (2010 est.)
Average Daily Caloric Consumption: 3,580
Adult Obesity Rate: 24% (2008)
Underweight Children under Age 5: Unknown or Negligible

Although the Portuguese eat a basically Mediterranean-style diet, it tends to be heavy in carbohydrates and sugar. Egg-based desserts are common, and a day's food intake may be more than what is required. The diet is varied, with adequate protein and vitamins from many vegetables and fruits. Although fish is eaten often, many Portuguese may consume excessive amounts of cholesterol from eggs and saturated fats in meats. Portugal's men have a lower rate of death by heart attacks than those in other European Union countries but a considerably higher rate of strokes.

Pamela Elder

Further Reading

Leite, David. *The New Portuguese Table.* New York: Clarkson Potter, 2009.

Robertson, Carol. *Portuguese Cooking: The Traditional Cuisine of Portugal.* Berkeley, CA: North Atlantic Books, 2008.

Romania

Population: 21,790,479 (July 2013 est.)
Population Rank: 56th
Population Growth Rate: −0.27% (2013 est.)
Life Expectancy at Birth: 74.45 years (2013 est.)
Health Expenditures: 5.9% of GDP (2010)
People with Access to Safe Drinking Water: 84% of population (2000 est.)
Average Daily Caloric Consumption: 3,510
Adult Obesity Rate: 19.1% (2008)
Underweight Children under Age 5: 3.5% (2002)

Many Romanians who lived through the Communist period and its aftermath know too well the close relationship between food and health. In the harshest years of the regime, food shortages were a part of daily life. Under the presidency of Nicolae Ceausescu from 1967 to 1989, money was being spent on the development of grand buildings, and food was being exported to pay off debt, while programs such as the Rational Nourishment Commission were implemented to hide the fact that there was not enough food for the nation. Understandably, today, many Romanians view health and nutrition campaigns with suspicion. The Communist period continued to influence health in Romania even after the expulsion of Ceausescu and the opening of Romania to a free-trade economy. From the early 1990s Romania had to completely rebuild systems of health care and food production and distribution. Subsidies that had been in place for many foods were removed. Real incomes were low, and food prices high. In the mid-1990s more than half the population lived below the poverty line, and many households spent as much as 70 percent of their income on food. All of this had a negative impact on the health of much of the Romanian population. Low life expectancies and high levels of diseases related to lifestyle have been reported for much of the period after the collapse of the Communist regime.

The situation today has largely improved. However, the health of Romanians, and people living in many other former Soviet states, is still below the European Union average, based on a number of health indicators. Diet plays an important part in this. Romania has registered a high number of diseases that relate to poverty and inadequate nutrition. Many studies indicate that poor diet and alcohol and tobacco consumption, particularly among men, have contributed to poor health in Romania. The high consumption of fats and oils and calories of low quality from the point of view of nutritional standards is likely to be a contributing factor.

Fruit and vegetable consumption in Romania has fluctuated and at times has been considerably lower than the recommended daily intake. This is partly due to issues of food scarcity and high prices and partly due to the style of the cuisine. While vegetable intake has increased in recent years, the percentage of potatoes that contribute to this has, too. The higher consumption of potatoes and cereals as major caloric items means that intake of many vitamins and minerals is reduced. Low fruit and vegetable intake, according to the World Health Organization, is one of the leading factors in many of the health issues faced by Romania today. However, the produce that is eaten is normally fresh, since much of it is produced locally, and it generally contains low levels of chemicals because of the high costs of herbicides and pesticides.

Kate Johnston

Mititei (Grilled Sausage Rolls)

Mititei is one of the most common Romanian foods. They can be served as part of a mezea, in the center of a mixed grill of meats, or as a main dish.

9 oz minced pork
9 oz minced beef
1 onion, finely chopped
2 garlic cloves, crushed
$\frac{1}{2}$ tsp baking powder
$\frac{1}{4}$ tsp thyme
1 tsp paprika
Salt and pepper
1 slice white bread, moistened with a little water
1 tbsp olive oil, for frying
3 tbsp chicken or vegetable stock

Combine all the ingredients, apart from the olive oil and stock, together in a large mixing bowl. Knead for about 5 minutes. The ingredients must be very well combined. Let the mixture sit for at least 1 hour. Divide the mixture into small handfuls, and roll into small sausage shapes. Brush with oil, and grill on a barbecue or fry in a pan for 10–15 minutes. Turn them several times during cooking, and baste with a little stock to keep them moist, if you like. Serve with pickled vegetables and salad or as an appetizer.

Further Reading

Kavena-Johnson, Maria. *Romania: The Melting Pot, Balkan Food and Cookery.* Totnes, Devon, UK: Prospect Books, 1999.

Sperber, Galia. *The Art of Romanian Cooking.* Gretna, LA: Pelican, 2002.

Russia

Population: 142,500,482 (July 2013 est.)
Population Rank: 9th
Population Growth Rate: –0.02% (2013 est.)
Life Expectancy at Birth: 69.85 years (2013 est.)
Health Expenditures: 6.2% of GDP (2011)

People with Access to Safe Drinking Water: 97% of population (2010 est.)
Average Daily Caloric Consumption: 3,270
Adult Obesity Rate: 26.5% (2008)
Underweight Children under Age 5: Unknown or Negligible

In Russia, food is not only treated as a source of nourishment and fuel but also valued for its preventative and curative role. Eating healthfully keeps a body fit and free of disease. Should they fall ill, Russians have numerous cures using a wide range of foods and medicinal herbs. The variety, purity, and freshness of food in Russia unfortunately are not enough to ensure proper health. Despite the conscious and continual efforts of mothers, wives, and grandmothers to feed and care for their families, health has generally deteriorated since 2000. Food, however, is only one part of the equation for good health.

Russians have several health-related problems in common: a short life expectancy, cardiovascular disease, and general nutritional deficiencies, as well as high rates of tobacco and alcohol use. Specific nutritional problems include the lack of affordability of certain healthful and essential food items, the suspect quality of some foodstuffs, and the absence of public awareness of what constitutes a healthful and balanced diet. Much of the overall decline in health, without a doubt, may be attributed to the social and economic disruptions since 1991. The Soviet experiment can be credited with improving the general diet of the lowest economic classes but not until well into the 1960s.

Quantity and freshness have priority over quality and finesse on the Russian table. Although restaurants and cafés are numerous in the big cities, hearty homemade meals are the ideal both in the countryside and in urban areas. A well-balanced meal should have a main course of fish or meat for flair, a starch (potatoes, pasta, or rice) for energy, and vegetables (often in the form of a cooked vegetable salad) for vitamins. Soup and tea are the bookends of a meal. Dessert would make it complete in the minds of most Russians. At least one hot meal a day is crucial to maintaining good digestion and health. Lunch, according to an earlier Russian tradition, was the main meal of the day. A light lunch is usually taken at work. The daily menu of most Russian families includes a meat or sausage dish. Therefore, the typical diet is very high in protein and animal fat, mostly from low-quality processed, smoked, or cured meats. Most people consume dairy products (usually fermented) daily, including cheese, dairy drinks (kefir, prostokvasha, *ryazhenka*), farmer's cheese (tvorog), and, more recently, yogurt. The most common vegetables are potatoes, cabbage, onions, tomatoes, and cucumbers.

Vegetables are almost always cooked (and often overcooked), except for tomatoes, cucumbers, and radishes, which are used in fresh salads.

Glenn R. Mack and Asele Surina

Further Reading

Mack, Glenn R., and Asele Surnia. *Food Culture in Russia and Central Asia.* Westport, CT: Greenwood Press, 2005.

Smith, R. E. F., and David Christian. *Bread and Salt: A Social and Economic History of Food and Drink in Russia.* Cambridge: Cambridge University Press, 1984.

Scotland

See Great Britain entry for statistical information

A strong social welfare system ensures that few in the United Kingdom go to bed hungry; however, a lack of education and cooking skills, and limited access to affordable, healthy food does mean that a significant portion of the

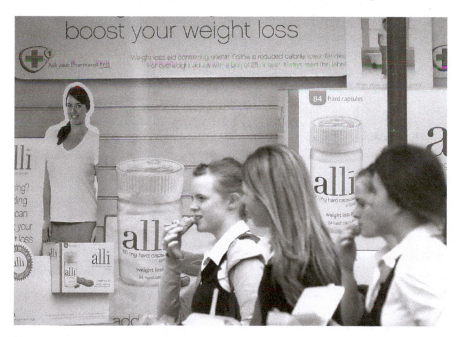

Scottish schoolgirls eat fast food while walking by advertisements for a weight-loss product. (Jeff J Mitchell/Getty Images)

population suffers from malnourishment. The government estimates that in 2005, 30 percent of patients admitted to hospitals or nursing homes were clinically malnourished. In Scotland specifically, eating habits are the second major cause of poor health after smoking.

Scotland's early industrialization not only made it more difficult for people to grow, store, and cook their own food but also altered people's understanding of their relationship to the land. The vestiges of that legacy are evident in the Scottish love of takeout, restaurants, and ready-made meals and in their penchant to eat quickly. An alarming number of Scots give set mealtimes or well-balanced meals little, if any, priority. People simply eat when they are hungry; they eat what tastes good, what is cheap, and what is readily available. While 40 percent of the Scottish population consumes fried food two or more times a week, a mere 10 percent eats whole wheat bread. Soft drink consumption has also gone up for both men and women. Younger Scots might have no more than a quick juice-type drink for breakfast, a package of crisps and a sausage for lunch, and a microwaved Scotch pie with chips for dinner, again with a soft drink or a beer.

An aggressive effort is under way to educate the public about the dangers of malnutrition and the importance of eating vegetables, fruit, lean meat, and whole grains. The 1991 white paper "Towards a Healthier Scotland" has set a number of goals aimed at stopping Scotland's rapidly increasing obesity and incidence of type 2 diabetes, including doubling its citizens' intake of whole-grain breads and whole-grain breakfast cereals, and consumption of fruits and vegetables.

Andrea Broomfield

Further Reading

Lawrence, Sue. *Cook's Tour of Scotland: From Barra to Brora in 120 Recipes.* London: Headline Books, 2006.

Wilson, Carol, and Christopher Trotter. *The Food and Cooking of Scotland.* London: Southwater, 2008.

Serbia

Population: 7,243,007 (July 2013 est.)
Population Rank: 98th
Population Growth Rate: –0.46% (2013 est.)
Life Expectancy at Birth: 74.79 years (2013 est.)
Health Expenditures: 10.4% of GDP (2011)

People with Access to Safe Drinking Water: 99% of population (2010 est.)
Average Daily Caloric Consumption: 2,710
Adult Obesity Rate: 24.8% (2008)
Underweight Children under Age 5: 1.8% (2006)

Since the early 1990s Serbia has undergone considerable demographic, economic, and nutritional transitions that compromised the population's food supply, especially for low-income socioeconomic groups. Reliable food production, processing, and distribution and food safety are real challenges in the development of the Serbian economy. Consequently, during the last decades many demographic, social, economic, and political changes influenced the food supply as well as dietary patterns in Serbia and resulted in a nutrition transition with an increase in the number of noncommunicable diseases. These have been the leading causes of morbidity, disability, and mortality for decades. The available data clearly indicate that smoking, hypertension, and physical inactivity as well as obesity are responsible for the greatest mortality burden, contributing 5.5 percent of total years of life lost in males and 7 percent in females. Diet represents one of the most relevant lifestyle risk factors contributing to the double burden of diet-related noncommunicable diseases. Overweight and obesity represent important public health challenge in Serbia.

Prevention of nutrition-related disorders is one of the major concerns of the Ministry of Health. There are several health-promotion and prevention programs in which regulation of body weight is an important issue; therefore prevention of overweight and obesity is included as one of the high-priority objectives. According to the findings of the 2006 Serbian Health Survey, based on the body mass index (BMI), 38.3 percent of adult Serbians had an optimum body weight, while one in two adults in Serbia was overweight or obese (54.5%), with 36.2 percent categorized as preobese and 18.3 percent as obese.

In 2005 the Ministry of Health set up an expert task force to develop the "Nutrition Action Plan for the Republic of Serbia." Key objectives of this action plan with respect to diet and health include ensuring a safe, healthy, and sustainable food supply and promoting healthy nutrition for all age groups. The key focus is to stop the increasing tendency toward obesity in children and adolescents, to eliminate micronutrient deficits across the population, and to monitor dietary habits.

The most frequent intestinal infectious diseases in 2006 in Serbia were diarrhea and gastroenteritis (44.55%) followed by bacterial intestinal infections (26.51%), bacterial alimentary intoxications (12.06%), and salmo-nellosis (9.41%)

Katrina Meynink

Cevapcici (Sausage)

1 lb minced lamb
1 lb minced pork
1 lb minced veal
3 cloves fresh garlic, peeled and finely chopped
1 large onion, peeled and finely chopped
Salt to taste
2 tbsp freshly ground black pepper
3 tbsp hot Hungarian paprika or sweet paprika
1 tsp freshly grated nutmeg

Mix together lamb, pork, veal, garlic, chopped onions, salt, and spices until thoroughly combined. Roll meat mixture into a long, ¾-inch cylinder. Cut links at 4-inch intervals. Or you can use a sausage extruder. Place on a plastic wrap–lined plate, cover with more plastic wrap, and refrigerate for 1 hour to firm. Panfry in a large nonstick frying pan for 8 minutes, turning frequently until brown on all sides.

Further Reading

Davies, Trish. *Cooking around the World: Romanian, Bulgarian and Balkan.* London: Lorenz Books, 2005.

Hawkesworth, Celia, trans. *Colović.* London: Hurst, 2002.

Slovenia

Population: 1,992,690 (July 2013 est.)
Population Rank: 147th
Population Growth Rate: –0.21% (2013 est.)
Life Expectancy at Birth: 77.66 years (2013 est.)
Health Expenditures: 9% of GDP (2010)
People with Access to Safe Drinking Water: 99% of population (2010 est.)
Average Daily Caloric Consumption: 3,220

Adult Obesity Rate: 28.6% (2008)
Underweight Children under Age 5: Unknown or Negligible

In the past centuries, the main preoccupation of the Slovene population was to ensure enough food, which, despite the meager means generally available for its purchase or cultivation, had to be prepared in a way that would provide enough energy for the heavy physical work that was required daily. Not much attention was paid to health or special diets. The two general exceptions were childbirth and severe illness. New mothers and the sick were given special food and beverages to restore their health as soon as possible so that they could return to work.

After a woman had given birth, her family had to provide adequate quantities of wine to renew her strength and vigor. The habit of giving wine to new mothers has been documented throughout the Slovene territory. She was also given a loaf of good white bread and a hen for hen soup, which was believed to possess special powers. Another dish recommended for new mothers and for those who were sick was the *tirjet*. It consisted of slices of white bread first dipped in wine and whisked egg and then fried.

Those who had problems with constipation were given pieces of dried pears or prunes soaked in water; equally recommendable were horseradish, which is a strong purgative, and lukewarm whey. Diarrhea was fought with dried huckleberries, dried pears, the *prežganka* (soup made from water and browned flour), and water in which unhusked wheat had been boiled for several hours.

Those who were anemic had to purify their blood with raw meat, particularly horse meat, fresh sauerkraut, and turnip shoots. Certain plants and vegetables, for example, dandelion, watercress, elder shoots, and wormwood buds, were believed to help as well. In case of dropsy, swooning, bronchial disease, nerves, and worms, folk medicine advised substantial quantities of garlic. Onions helped cure pulmonary diseases, colds, and rheumatism.

Today, interest in a healthy diet has increased primarily due to a growing number of articles in the printed and electronic media. According to experts, Slovenes consume too much fat, sugar, pork, and alcohol and too little fruit and vegetables. In view of this, the Ministry of Health has organized different activities and programs to promote the consumption of fruit, vegetables, and unsaturated fats.

Maja Godina-Golija

Further Reading

Bogataj, Janez. "The Festive Table." In *Culinary Cultures of Europe: Identity, Diversity and Dialogue*, edited by Darra Goldstein and Kathrin Merkle, 397–441. Strasbourg, France: Council of Europe Publishing, 2005.

Bogataj, Janez. *Taste Slovenia*. Washington, DC: National Geographic, 2007.

Spain

Population: 47,370,542 (July 2013 est.)
Population Rank: 28th
Population Growth Rate: 0.73% (2013 est.)
Life Expectancy at Birth: 81.37 years (2013 est.)
Health Expenditures: 9.6% of GDP (2010)
People with Access to Safe Drinking Water: 100% of population (2010 est.)
Average Daily Caloric Consumption: 3,270
Adult Obesity Rate: 26.6% (2008)
Underweight Children under Age 5: Unknown or Negligible

Much of Spain would until recent decades have been included among those people who ate a so-called Mediterranean diet, consisting of a small amount of animal protein, many fruits and vegetables, healthy oils (predominantly olive), and fish high in omega-3 fatty acids. This was not the case for mountainous parts of Spain and in particular the north, but in general the Spanish diet was parsimonious and healthy, though political turmoil certainly did add its share of poverty and malnutrition. With economic prosperity, Spain

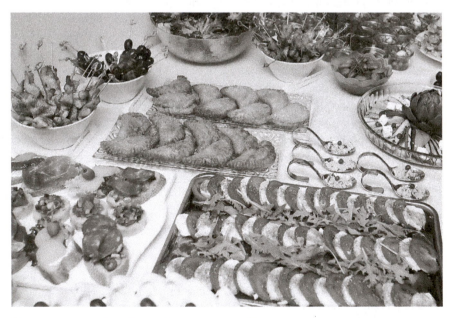

An assortment of traditional Spanish tapas. (Shutterstock)

can now be said to share with other nations the problems of hypertension, obesity, diabetes, and a diet relatively high in saturated fat, salt, and processed sugar. Cardiovascular disease is on the rise. This is compounded by an increasingly sedentary lifestyle, with people working at desks in an increasingly service economy and fewer people performing manual labor. Even agriculture, which a mere generation ago would have been physically very demanding, has been mechanized on par with industrial-scale farming in the wealthiest of countries. Ironically, the Spanish are also increasingly health conscious, and manufactured foods specifically designed for maintaining an ideal body weight, as well as low-calorie and low-cholesterol foods, are now commonly seen in grocery stores.

Ken Albala

Further Reading

Andres, Jose. *Made in Spain: Spanish Dishes for the American Kitchen.* New York: Clarkson Potter, 2008.

von Bremzen, Anya. *The New Spanish Table.* New York: Workman, 2005.

Sweden

Population: 9,119,423 (July 2013 est.)
Population Rank: 92nd
Population Growth Rate: 0.18% (2013 est.)
Life Expectancy at Birth: 81.28 years (2013 est.)
Health Expenditures: 9.4% of GDP (2011)
People with Access to Safe Drinking Water: 100% of population (2010 est.)
Average Daily Caloric Consumption: 3,170
Adult Obesity Rate: 18.6% (2008)
Underweight Children under Age 5: Unknown or Negligible

Swedes are very health conscious; many work out regularly and make mindful choices about the foods they eat. A lot of people are vegetarians or vegan, and others avoid red meat and pork. Recently, eating foods with a low glycemic index has become very popular, and many restaurants now offer at least one dish with a low glycemic index.

A few years ago, a journalist published a book about additives and preservatives, and Swedes were shocked about the high content of unnatural ingredients in their favorite foods. Therefore many Swedes now check the ingredients on packaged foods and try to avoid those they do not consider natural. A chain of supermarkets has taken advantage of this trend and is now marking "real food" to make it easier for their customers to find more natural products.

Another important trend is the strong movement toward organic and locally produced foods, which takes up a large part of the media discussions. Many cookbooks that deal with organic, regional, local, and unprocessed foods are published every year in Sweden. Food blogs are also very popular, and there are several that have organic and natural food as their favorite subject.

Sweden has a strong rural tradition, and many Swedes have a passion for nature and everything related to growing and cultivating plants. In many cities people may rent a small patch of land for growing their own food, and it is common for those who do to spend several days at a time in their lots, which most often have a small shed in which to spend the night. Recently, growers have organized small local markets, which have become very popular, in which they sell their surplus. Many who do not have access to arable land grow vegetables and even fruits at home, and it is common to see balconies in Sweden overflowing with cherry tomato plants and different kinds of herbs.

Gabriela Villagran Backman

Further Reading

Mosesson, Anna. *Swedish Food and Cooking: Traditions, Ingredients, Tastes, Techniques, over 60 Classic Recipes.* London: Aquamarine, 2006.

Notaker, Henry. *Food Culture in Scandinavia.* Westport, CT: Greenwood Press, 2008.

Switzerland

Population: 7,996,026 (July 2013 est.)
Population Rank: 95th
Population Growth Rate: 0.85% (2013 est.)
Life Expectancy at Birth: 82.28 years (2013 est.)
Health Expenditures: 10.9% of GDP (2011)
People with Access to Safe Drinking Water: 100% of population (2010 est.)
Average Daily Caloric Consumption: 3,420
Adult Obesity Rate: 17.5% (2008)
Underweight Children under Age 5: Unknown or Negligible

Like many European countries, Switzerland has seen its obesity rate rise over the last 20 years. According to the Federal Office of Public Health,

37.3 percent of Swiss adults have a body mass index greater than 25, which makes them overweight. One out of five children is overweight—a number that has quintupled in 20 years. A decline in physical activity, as both work and leisure become more sedentary, and a diet of high-calorie foods rich in fats and sugars are to blame.

Generally, however, the Swiss lifestyle offers a better work-life balance than other Western countries. While freelancing is not very common, employees can often reduce their work schedule once they start having children or to pursue side activities. Having more time at home means that people cook full meals and bake often. Even the larger cities are close to mountains and lakes, so outdoor activities are part of the everyday life of most Swiss citizens, from a simple walk or a multiday hike at high altitude to boating and skiing.

Grains and dairy products appear frequently on Swiss tables, as do vegetables. Because of its cost, meat is typically not consumed daily. Many still take the time to sit down for breakfast, which includes muesli or bread slices with jams rather than sweet pastries. This makes the Swiss diet a generally balanced one.

Anne Engammare McBride

Cheese Fondue

Serves 4

If you are a real garlic lover, you can also add a clove—thinly sliced or finely minced—to the fondue itself, for a more pronounced taste.

1 clove garlic
1/4 tsp cornstarch
2/3 lb Gruyère, cut in small cubes or grated
2/3 lb Vacherin, cut in small pieces (or substitute a soft, ripe cow-milk cheese)
1/3 c dry white wine, preferably Fendant
1 tbsp kirsch or more to taste
Freshly ground white pepper
Plenty of thick-crusted peasant bread, torn or cut in pieces

Rub an earthenware fondue pot with the garlic clove.

Dissolve the cornstarch in a couple of tablespoons of the wine. Place the Gruyère and Vacherin in the pot, and add the wine, the dissolved cornstarch, and the kirsch.

Place the pot on the stovetop over medium-low heat, and stir with a wooden spoon until the cheese melts and everything forms a homogeneous mixture.

Light a container of Sterno canned heat or chafing gel, and place in the appropriate receptacle in the fondue burner stand. Place the fondue pot on the stand. Make sure that the cheese does not come to a boil. You can control the heat dispersed by turning the cover of the burner to open or close its ventilation holes.

Dip the pieces of bread into the fondue by placing them on long-handled forks.

Further Reading

Bossi, Betty. *Cuisine Suisse*. Zurich: Editions Betty Bossi, 2009.

Nelson, Kay Shaw. *Cuisines of the Alps: Recipes, Drinks, and Lore from France, Switzerland, Liechtenstein, Italy, Germany, Austria, and Slovenia*. New York: Hippocrene Books, 2005.

Weiss, Martin. *Urchuchi: Schweizer Restaurants mit Geschichten und Gerichten*. Zurich: Rotpunktverlag, 2007–9.

Ukraine

Population: 44,573,205 (July 2013 est.)
Population Rank: 30th
Population Growth Rate: –0.63% (2013 est.)
Life Expectancy at Birth: 68.93 years (2013 est.)
Health Expenditures: 7.3% of GDP (2011)
People with Access to Safe Drinking Water: 98% of population (2010 est.)
Average Daily Caloric Consumption: 3,230
Adult Obesity Rate: 21.3% (2008)
Underweight Children under Age 5: 0.9% (2002)

Many younger Ukrainians see the traditional Ukrainian diet of starchy foods along with fatty pork as unhealthy. Today, the population of Ukraine, like that of the rest of Europe, is heavily urbanized. The traditional diet, created to restore the strength of people engaged in heavy farm labor, is no longer relevant to modern work and life. Indeed, in the twentieth century, a diet rich in fat and carbohydrates, along with industrial pollution, heavy smoking, and drinking, has contributed to a rise in cardiovascular disease among Ukrainians. Ukrainians also argue that the traditional diet was varied and natural and should be retained instead of consuming industrially processed and imported foods. Pollution from the 1986 nuclear disaster at Chernobyl is also a major concern.

Ukrainians retain many traditional folk remedies for various disorders, as modern medicine is poorly funded and often seen as corrupt. Herbal teas are used to soothe a system out of order. Chamomile tea is used in case of a stomachache. Black tea with honey and lemon is used to soothe sore throats. Alcohol, honey, garlic, and even hot milk are seen as medicinal for many respiratory disorders. Strong-smelling herbs and garlic have been seen as not only medicinal but also useful for scaring away evil spirits. These beliefs have been retained in the Ukrainian countryside and were resurrected after the fall of the Soviet Union.

Anton Masterovoy

Further Reading

Ponomarenko, Ninel. *Taste of My Ukrainian Homeland.* Westfield, Tunbridge Wells, UK: Upso, 2004.

Zahny, Bodan. *The Best of Ukrainian Cuisine.* New York: Hippocrene Books, 1998.

Other

Antarctica

Because of the extreme Antarctic climate, early rations were more than double the recommended daily dietary intake: about 4,700 calories (Swithinbank 1997). Now that many researchers spend the majority of their time indoors, efforts are made to provide lower-calorie, healthy meals as well as ample opportunities for physical exercise, especially in the dark winter when it is nearly impossible to venture outdoors.

Early explorers suffered from scurvy and vitamin A toxicity (hypervitaminosis A) due to a diet based on seal and penguin (high in vitamin A, especially the liver) with few or no fruits or vegetables. This caused a loss of hair and teeth and skin lesions. Starvation and extreme hunger were constant concerns—and the unfortunate end—of many early Antarctic explorers.

While many tend to view gastronomic variety as a luxury, there seems to be evidence that in times of scarcity, thought of food can be psychologically debilitating if left untended. Mawson and his colleagues wrote extensive menus while subsisting on dog through an Antarctic trek. "Young duck with apple sauce, *petit pois,* new potatoes and American sweet corn" are some of the 11 courses they devise for their return home to Sydney, Australia (Jacka and Jacka 1988, 39).

Similarly elaborate food dreams abound in the early Antarctic literature, characterized by an abundance of food and a rude awakening when the dreamer discovers it is unattainable. Mawson dreamed of buying an elaborate cake in a confectioner's shop and accidentally leaving the store without the cake. When he returned, the shop had a sign in the door that read "early closing" (Jacka and Jacka 1988, 175–76).

Wilson writes of dreams with unnerving similarity to Mawson's:

Nearly every night we dream of eating and food. Very hungry always, our allowance being a bare one. Dreams as a rule of splendid food, ball suppers, sirloins of beef, cauldrons full of steaming vegetables. But one spends all one's time shouting at waiters who won't bring one a plate of anything, or else one finds the beef is only ashes when one gets it, or a pot full of honey has been poured out on a sawdusty floor. One very rarely gets a feed in one's sleep, though occasionally one does. For one night I dreamed that I eat the whole of a large cake in the hall at Westal without thinking and was horribly ashamed when I realized it had been put there for a drawing room tea, and everyone was asking where the cake was gone. These dreams are very vivid, I remember them now, though it is two months since I dreamed them. (Savours 1966/1904, 221)

Because of the diversity of the research station personnel and the international treaty managing the continent, all of the world's major religions are represented on the continent at one time or another. There are particular challenges for researchers who require a vegetarian, halal, or kosher diet, and extensive arrangements need to be made in advance since food deliveries to the stations are infrequent and other options for dining do not exist.

In considering the food of Antarctica, past and present, two themes emerge. The first is the idea that food is a necessary burden that needs to be handled deftly and efficiently in order to make for a successful expedition, be it one of early exploration or present-day research. The second theme is that despite the inhospitable climate and geography of the continent, there is a need to occasionally eschew efficiency and practicality to feed the nostalgic, impractical impulses of the resident. These two themes synthesize to form a contemporary Antarctic food culture that is neither wanton nor ascetic and that prides itself on improvisation, making the most of that which is available. In the words of Sir Douglas Mawson, it is "a subject ... which requires particular consideration and study" (1998/1911, 115).

Jonathan Deutsch

Further Reading

Subramanian, V., and T. R. Sharma. "Processed Food on Antarctica." *Indian Food Industry* 3, No. 3 (1982–84): 99–100.

Wheeler, Sara. *Terra Incognita: Travels in Antarctica.* London: Jonathan Cape, 1996.

Space

Health is a primary concern on all space missions, and every facet of the astronaut's physiology and metabolism is scrupulously monitored, especially given the unique circumstances of weightlessness and the tendency to lose muscle mass and experience other forms of fatigue. The dietary composition of space food is likewise carefully analyzed by nutritionists and naturally changes with the development of nutritional science over the decades since humans were first sent into space.

Jane Levi

Gemini Mashed Potatoes

Most of the processing of space food demands industrial techniques that are impossible to replicate domestically. The keen experimenter is limited to using common foods available in the local supermarket and attempting to replicate the space experience by improvising appropriate packaging.

1 package dehydrated mashed potatoes
1 ziplock bag with label
1 syringe
Cold water (quantity according to instructions on original package)

Carefully tip the dehydrated potatoes into the ziplock bag. Seal the bag. Measure the water into the syringe. Inject water into the bag, as close to the seal as possible. Gently massage the bag until the water is evenly distributed and the potato is hydrated. Open one corner of the package and eat with a teaspoon.

Further Reading
Bourland, Charles T., and Gregory L. Vogt. *The Astronaut's Cookbook: Tales, Recipes and More*. New York: Springer, 2009.

About the Editor and Contributors

Editor

KEN ALBALA is Professor of History at the University of the Pacific in Stockton, California. He is the author or editor of seventeen books including *Eating Right in the Renaissance* and *The Banquet and Beans: A History*. He has also coauthored two cookbooks: *The Lost Art of Real Cooking* and *The Lost Arts of Hearth and Home*. Albala was editor of ABC-CLIO/Greenwood's *Food Culture around the World* series with 29 volumes in print.

Contributors

JULIA ABRAMSON has visited France on a regular basis for more than twenty five years to study, research, travel, and eat. She has published essays on aspects of food culture from vegetable carving to gastronomic writing and is the author of the book *Food Culture in France*. Abramson teaches French literature and culture and food studies at the University of Oklahoma, Norman.

M. SHAHRIM AL-KARIM is a senior lecturer of food service and hospitality management at the Universiti Putra Malaysia. His research interests include food and culture, culinary tourism, food habits, and consumer behavior. He received a BS in hotel and restaurant management from New York University; an MBA from Universiti Teknologi MARA, Malaysia; and a PhD in hospitality and tourism from Oklahoma State University, United States.

E. N. ANDERSON is professor emeritus of the Department of Anthropology, University of California, Riverside.

LAURA P. APPELL-WARREN holds a doctorate in psychological anthropology from Harvard University. Her primary focus of research has been the study of personhood; however, she has also studied the effects of social change on children's play. She has done research among the Bulusu' of East Kalimantan, Indonesia, and among the Rungus Momogon, a Dusunic-speaking peoples, of Sabah, Malaysia. In addition, she has traveled widely throughout Arctic Canada. She is the editor of *The Iban Diaries of Monica Freeman 1949–1951: Including Ethnographic Drawings, Sketches, Paintings, Photographs and Letters* and is author of the forthcoming volume entitled *Personhood: An Examination of the History and Use of an Anthropological Concept.* In addition to her current research on cradleboard use among Native North Americans, she is a teacher of anthropology at St. Mark's School in Southborough, Massachusetts.

HEATHER ARNDT-ANDERSON is a Portland, Oregon, native who draws culinary inspiration from many world cuisines but prefers cooking from her own backyard. She is a part-time natural resources consultant and a full-time radical homemaker; in her (rare) spare time she writes the food blog *Voodoo & Sauce.*

MICHAEL ASHKENAZI is a scholar, writer, and consultant who has been researching and writing about Japanese food since 1990. In addition to books and articles on Japanese society, including its food culture, he has written numerous scholarly and professional articles and papers on various subjects including theoretical and methodological issues in anthropology, organized violence, space exploration, migration, religion and ritual, resettling ex-combatants, and small arms. He has taught at higher-education institutions in Japan, Canada, Israel, and the United Kingdom, directing graduate and undergraduate students. He is currently senior researcher and project leader at the Bonn International Center for Conversion in Germany, with responsibility for the areas of small arms and reintegration of ex-combatants. He has conducted field research in East and Southeast Asia, East and West Africa, the Middle East, and Latin America.

BABETTE AUDANT went to Prague after college, where she quickly gave up teaching English in order to cook at a classical French restaurant. After graduating from the Culinary Institute of America, she worked as a chef in New York City for eight years, working at the Rainbow Room, Beacon Bar & Grill, and other top-rated restaurants. She is a lecturer at City University of New York

Kingsborough's Department of Tourism and Hospitality, and a doctoral candidate in geography at the City University of New York Graduate Center. Her research focuses on public markets and food policy in New York City.

GABRIELA VILLAGRAN BACKMAN, MA (English and Hispanic literature), was born in Sweden and raised in Mexico and the United States; she currently lives in Stockholm, Sweden. She is an independent researcher, interested in food studies, cultural heritage, writing cookbooks, red wine, and the Internet.

CAROLYN BÁNFALVI is a writer based in Budapest. She is the author of *Food Wine Budapest* (Little Bookroom) and *The Food and Wine Lover's Guide to Hungary: With Budapest Restaurants and Trips to the Wine Country* (Park Kiado). She contributes to numerous international food and travel publications and leads food and wine tours through Taste Hungary, her culinary tour company.

PETER BARRETT is a painter who writes a food blog and is also the Food & Drink writer for *Chronogram Magazine* in New York's Hudson Valley.

CYNTHIA D. BERTELSEN is an independent culinary scholar, nutritionist, freelance food writer, and food columnist. She lived in Haiti for three years and worked on a food-consumption study for a farming-systems project in Jacmel, Haiti. She writes a food history blog, *Gherkins & Tomatoes,* found at http://gherkinstomatoes.com.

MEGAN K. BLAKE is a senior lecturer in geography at the University of Sheffield. She has published research that examines the intersections between place and social practices. While her previous work focused on entrepreneurship and innovation, her recent work has examined food practices and family life.

ANDREA BROOMFIELD is associate professor of English at Johnson County Community College in Overland Park, Kansas, and author of *Food and Cooking in Victorian England: A History.*

CYNTHIA CLAMPITT is a culinary historian, world traveler, and award-winning author. In 2010, she was elected to the Society of Women Geographers.

NEIL L. COLETTA is assistant director of food, wine, and the arts and lecturer in the MLA in gastronomy program at Boston University. His current research includes food and aesthetics and experimental pedagogy in the field of food studies.

PAUL CRASK is a travel writer and the author of two travel guides: *Dominica* (2008) and *Grenada, Carriacou and Petite Martinique* (2009).

CHRISTINE CRAWFORD-OPPENHEIMER is the information services librarian and archivist at the Culinary Institute of America. She grew up in Ras Tanura, Saudi Arabia.

ANITA VERNA CROFTS is on the faculty at the University of Washington's Department of Communication, where she serves as an associate director of the master of communication in digital media program. In addition, she holds an appointment at the University of Washington's Department of Global Health, where she collaborates with partner institutions in Sudan, Namibia, and India on trainings that address leadership, management, and policy development, with her contributions targeted at the concept of storytelling as a leadership and evidence tool. Anita is an intrepid chowhound and publishes on gastroethnographic topics related to the intersection of food and identity. She hosts the blog *Sneeze!* at her website http://www.pepperforthebeast.com.

LIZA DEBEVEC is a research fellow at the Scientific Research Centre of the Slovene Academy of sciences and arts in Ljubljana, Slovenia. She has a PhD in social anthropology from the University of St. Andrews, United Kingdom. Her research interests are West Africa and Burkina Faso, food studies, Islam, gender, identity, and practice of everyday life.

JONATHAN DEUTSCH is associate professor of culinary arts at Kingsborough Community College, City University of New York, and Public Health, City University of New York Graduate Center. He is the author or editor of five books including, with Sarah Billingsley, *Culinary Improvisation* (Pearson, 2010) and, with Annie Hauck-Lawson, *Gastropolis: Food and New York City* (Columbia University Press, 2009).

DEBORAH DUCHON is a nutritional anthropologist in Atlanta, Georgia.

NATHALIE DUPREE is the author of ten cookbooks, many of which are about the American South, for which she has won two James Beard Awards. She has hosted over 300 television shows on the Public Broadcasting Service, the Food Network, and TLC. She lives with her husband, Jack Bass, who has authored 9 books about the American South and helped with her contribution to *Food Cultures of the World*.

PAMELA ELDER has worked in food public relations and online culinary education and is a freelance writer in the San Francisco Bay area.

RACHEL FINN is a freelance writer whose work has appeared in various print and online publications. She is the founder and director of Roots Cuisine, a nonprofit organization dedicated to promoting the food-ways of the African diaspora around the globe.

RICHARD FOSS has been a food writer and culinary historian since 1986, when he started as a restaurant critic for the *Los Angeles Reader*. His book on the history of rum is slated for publication in 2011, to be followed by a book on the history of beachside dining in Los Angeles. He also is a science fiction and fantasy author, an instructor in culinary history and Elizabethan theater at the University of California, Los Angeles, Extension, and on the board of the Culinary Historians of Southern California.

NANCY G. FREEMAN is a food writer and art historian living in Berkeley, California, with a passion for food history. She has written about cuisines ranging from Ethiopia to the Philippines to the American South.

RAMIN GANESHRAM is a veteran journalist and professional chef trained at the Institute of Culinary Education in New York City, where she has also worked as a recreational chef instructor. Ganeshram also holds a master's degree in journalism from Columbia University. For eight years she worked as a feature writer/stringer for the *New York Times* regional sections, and she spent another eight years as a food columnist and feature writer for *Newsday*. She is the author of *Sweet Hands: Island Cooking from Trinidad and Tobago* (Hippocrene, 2006; 2nd expanded edition, 2010) and *Stir It Up* (Scholastic, 2011). In addition to contributing to a variety of food publications including *Saveur, Gourmet, Bon Appetit*, and epicurious.com, Ganeshram has written articles on food, culture, and travel for *Islands* (as contributing editor),

National Geographic Traveler, Forbes Traveler, Forbes Four Seasons, and many others. Currently, Ganeshram teaches food writing for New York University's School of Continuing Professional Studies.

HANNA GARTH is a doctoral candidate in the Department of Anthropology at the University of California, Los Angeles. She is currently working on a dissertation on household food practices in Santiago de Cuba. Previously, she has conducted research on food culture, health, and nutrition in Cuba, Chile, and the Philippines.

MARY GEE is a medical sociology doctoral student at the University of California, San Francisco. Her current research interests include herbalism and Asian and Asian American foodways, especially with regard to multigenerational differences. Since 1995, she has actively worked with local and national eating disorders research and policy and advocacy organizations as well as for a program evaluation research consulting firm.

CHE ANN ABDUL GHANI holds a bachelor's degree in English and a master's degree in linguistics. She has a keen interest in studying language and language use in gastronomy. She is currently attached to the English Department at Universiti Putra Malaysia. Her research interests range from the use of language in context (pragmatics) to language use in multidisciplinary areas, namely, disciplines related to the social sciences. She also carries out work in translation and editing.

MAJA GODINA-GOLIJA is research advisor at the Institute of Slovenian Ethnology, Scientific Research Centre of Slovenian Academy of Science and Arts, Ljubljana, Slovenia.

ANNIE GOLDBERG is a graduate student studying gastronomy at Boston University.

DARRA GOLDSTEIN is Frances Christopher Oakley Third Century Professor of Russian at Williams College and the founding editor-in-chief of *Gastronomica: The Journal of Food and Culture*.

KEIKO GOTO, PhD, is associate professor at the Department of Nutrition and Food Sciences, California State University, Chico. Dr. Goto has more than fifteen years of work experience in the field of nutrition and has worked as a practitioner and researcher in various developing countries. Dr. Goto's current research areas include food and culture, child and adolescent nutrition, sustainable food systems, and international nutrition.

CARLA GUERRÓN MONTERO is a cultural and applied anthropologist trained in Latin America and the United States. She is currently associate professor of anthropology in the Department of Anthropology at the University of Delaware. Dr. Guerrón Montero's areas of expertise include gender, ethnicity, and identity; processes of globalization/nationalism, and particularly tourism; and social justice and human rights.

MARY GUNDERSON calls her practice paleocuisineology, where food and cooking bring cultures alive. Through many media, including the sites HistoryCooks.com and MaryGunderson.com, she writes and speaks about South and North American food history and contemporary creative living and wellness. She wrote and published the award-winning book *The Food Journal of Lewis and Clark: Recipes for an Expedition* (History Cooks, 2003) and has authored six food-history books for kids.

LIORA GVION is a senior lecturer at the Kibbutzim College of Education and also teaches at the Faculty of Agriculture, Food and Environment at the Institute of Biochemistry, Food Science and Nutrition Hebrew University of Jerusalem.

CHERIE Y. HAMILTON is a cookbook author and specialist on the food cultures and cuisines of the Portuguese-speaking countries in Europe, South America, Africa, and Asia.

JESSICA B. HARRIS teaches English at Queens College/City University of New York and is director of the Institute for the Study of Culinary Cultures at Dillard University.

MELANIE HAUPT is a doctoral candidate in English at the University of Texas at Austin. Her dissertation, "Starting from Scratch: Reading Women's Cooking Communities," explores women's use of cookbooks and recipes in the formation and reification of real and virtual communities.

URSULA HEINZELMANN is an independent scholar and culinary historian, twice awarded the prestigious Sophie Coe Prize. A trained chef, sommelier, and ex-restaurateur, she now works as a freelance wine and food writer and journalist based in Berlin, Germany.

JENNIFER HOSTETTER is an independent food consultant specializing in writing, research, and editing. She has degrees in history and culinary arts and holds a master's degree in food culture and communications from the University of Gastronomic Sciences in Italy. She also served as editorial assistant for this encyclopedia.

KELILA JAFFE is a doctoral candidate in the Food Studies Program at New York University. Originally from Sonoma, California, and the daughter of a professional chef, she has pursued anthropological and archaeological food-ways research since her entry into academia. She received a BA with distinction in anthropology from the University of Pennsylvania, before attending the University of Auckland, where she earned an MA with honors in anthropology, concentrating in archaeology. Her research interests include past foodways, domestication, and zooarchaeology, and she has conducted fieldwork in Fiji, New Zealand, and Hawaii.

ZILKIA JANER is associate professor of global studies at Hofstra University in New York. She is the author of *Puerto Rican Nation-Building Literature: Impossible Romance* (2005) and *Latino Food Culture* (2008).

BRELYN JOHNSON is a graduate of the master's program in food studies at New York University.

KATE JOHNSTON is currently based in Italy, where she is an independent cultural food researcher and writer and a daily ethnographer of people's food habits. She has a degree in anthropology from Macquarie University in Sydney, Australia, and a recent master's degree in food culture and communication from the University of Gastronomic Sciences, Italy. She was also editorial assistant for this encyclopedia.

DESIREE KOH was born and raised in Singapore. A writer focusing on travel, hospitality, sports, fitness, business, and, of course, food, Koh's explorations across the globe always begin at the market, as she believes that the sight, scent, and savoring of native produce and cuisine are the key to the city's heart. The first and only female in Major League Eating's Asia debut,

Koh retired from competition to better focus on each nibble and sip of fine, hopefully slow food.

BRUCE KRAIG is emeritus professor of history at Roosevelt University in Chicago and adjunct faculty at the Culinary School of Kendall College, Chicago. He has published and edited widely in the field of American and world food history. Kraig is also the founding president of the Culinary Historians of Chicago and the Greater Midwest Foodways Alliance.

R. J. KRAJEWSKI is the research services librarian at Simmons College, where among other things he facilitates discovery of food-culture research, especially through the lens of race, class, and gender. His own engagement with food is seasonally and locally rooted, starting in his own small, urban homestead, much like his Polish and German ancestors.

ERIN LAVERTY is a freelance food writer and researcher based in Brooklyn, New York. She holds a master's degree in food studies from New York University.

ROBERT A. LEONARD has a PhD in theoretical linguistics from Columbia. He studies the way people create and communicate meaning, including through food. He was born in Brooklyn and trained as a cook and *panaderia-reposteria* manager in the Caribbean; his doctoral studies led him to eight years of fieldwork in language, culture, and food in Africa and Southeast Asia. In the arts, as an undergraduate he cofounded and led the rock group Sha Na Na and with them opened for their friend Jimi Hendrix at the Woodstock Festival. Leonard is probably one of a very few people who have worked with both the Grateful Dead and the Federal Bureau of Investigation, which in recent years recruited him to teach the emerging science of forensic linguistics at Quantico.

JANE LEVI is an independent consultant and writer based in London, England. She is currently working on her PhD at the London Consortium, examining food in utopias, funded by her work on posttrade financial policy in the City of London.

YRSA LINDQVIST is a European ethnologist working as the leading archivist at the Folk Culture Archive in Helsinki. Her research about food and eating habits in the late 1990s, combined with earlier collections at the archive, resulted in 2009 in the publication *Mat, Måltid, Minne.· Hundraår av finlandssvensk matkulur.* The book analyzes the changes in housekeeping and attitudes toward food. She has also contributed to other publications focusing on identity questions and has worked as a junior researcher at the Academy of Finland.

WILLIAM G. LOCKWOOD is professor emeritus of cultural anthropology at the University of Michigan. His central interest is ethnicity and interethnic relations. He has conducted long-term field research in Bosnia-Herzegovina and the Croatian community in Austria and also among Roma and with a variety of ethnic groups in America, including Arabs, Finns, and Bosnians. He has long held a special interest in how food functions in ethnic group maintenance and in reflecting intra-and intergroup relations.

YVONNE R. LOCKWOOD is curator emeritus of folklife at the Michigan State University Museum. Her formal training is in folklore, history, and Slavic languages and literatures. Research in Bosnia, Austria, and the United States, especially the Great Lakes region, has resulted in numerous publications, exhibitions, festival presentations, and workshops focused on her primary interests of foodways and ethnic traditions.

JANET LONG-SOLÍS, an anthropologist and archaeologist, is a research associate at the Institute of Historical Research at the National University of Mexico. She has published several books and articles on the chili pepper, the history of Mexican food, and the exchange of food products between Europe and the Americas in the sixteenth century.

KRISTINA LUPP has a background in professional cooking and has worked in Toronto and Florence. She is currently pursuing a master of arts in gastronomy at the University of Adelaide.

MÁIRTÍN MAC CON IOMAIRE is a lecturer in culinary arts in the Dublin Institute of Technology. Máirtín is well known as a chef, culinary historian, food writer, broadcaster, and ballad singer. He lives in Dublin with his wife and two daughters. He was the first Irish chef to be awarded a PhD, for his oral history of Dublin restaurants.

GLENN R. MACK is a food historian with extensive culinary training in Uzbekistan, Russia, Italy, and the United States. He cofounded the Culinary

Academy of Austin and the Historic Foodways Group of Austin and currently serves as president of Le Cordon Bleu College of Culinary Arts Atlanta.

ANDREA MACRAE is a lecturer in the Le Cordon Bleu Graduate Program in Gastronomy at the University of Adelaide, Australia.

GIORGOS MALTEZAKIS earned his PhD in anthropology with research in cooperation with the Institute Studiorium Humanitatis of the Ljubljana Graduate School of the Humanities. His dissertation was on consumerism, the global market, and food, which was an ethnographic approach to the perception of food in Greece and Slovenia.

BERTIE MANDELBLATT is assistant professor at the University of Toronto, cross-appointed to the departments of Historical Studies and Geography. Her research concerns the early-modern French Atlantic, with a focus on commodity exchanges at the local and global scales: Her two current projects are the history of food provisioning in the Franco-Caribbean and the transatlantic circulation of French rum and molasses, in both the seventeenth and eighteenth centuries.

MARTY MARTINDALE is a freelance writer living in Largo, Florida.

LAURA MASON is a writer and food historian with a special interest in local, regional, and traditional foods in the United Kingdom and elsewhere. Her career has explored many dimensions of food and food production, including cooking for a living, unraveling the history of sugar confectionery, and trying to work out how many traditional and typically British foods relate to culture and landscape. Her publications include *Taste of Britain* (with Catherine Brown; HarperCollins, 2006), *The Food Culture of Great Britain* (Greenwood, 2004), and *The National Trust Farmhouse Cookbook* (National Trust, 2009).

ANTON MASTEROVOY is a PhD candidate at the Graduate Center, City University of New York. He is working on his dissertation, titled "Eating Soviet: Food and Culture in USSR, 1917–1991."

ANNE ENGAMMARE MCBRIDE, a Swiss native, food writer, and editor, is the director of the Experimental Cuisine Collective and a food studies PhD candidate at New York University. Her most recent book is *Culinary Careers: How to Get Your Dream Job in Food*, coauthored with Rick Smilow.

MICHAEL R. MCDONALD is associate professor of anthropology at Florida Gulf Coast University. He is the author of *Food Culture in Central America*.

NAOMI M. MCPHERSON is associate professor of cultural anthropology and graduate program coordinator at the University of British Columbia, Okanagan Campus. Since 1981, she has accumulated over three years of field research with the Bariai of West New Britain, Papua New Guinea.

KATRINA MEYNINK is an Australia-based freelance food writer and researcher. She has a master's degree in gastronomy through Le Cordon Bleu and the University of Adelaide under a scholarship from the James Beard Foundation. She is currently completing her first cookbook.

BARBARA J. MICHAEL is a sociocultural anthropologist whose research focuses on social organization, economics, decision making, and gender. Her geographic focus is on the Middle East and East Africa, where she has done research with the pastoral nomadic Hawazma Baggara and on traditional medicine in Yemen and is working on a video about men's cafes as a social institution. She teaches anthropology at the University of North Carolina, Wilmington, and has also worked as a consultant for several United Nations agencies.

DIANA MINCYTE is a fellow at the Rachel Carson Center at the Ludwig Maximilian University, Munich, and visiting assistant professor in the Department of Advertising at the University of Illinois, Urbana-Champaign. Mincyte examines topics at the interface of food, the environment, risk society, and global inequalities. Her book investigates raw-milk politics in the European Union to consider the production risk society and its institutions in post-Socialist states.

REBECCA MOORE is a doctoral student studying the history of biotechnology at the University of Toronto in Ontario, Canada.

NAWAL NASRALLAH, a native of Iraq, was a professor of English and comparative literature at the universities of Baghdad and Mosul until 1990. As an independent scholar, she wrote the award-winning *Delights from the Garden of Eden: A Cookbook and a History of the Iraqi Cuisine* and *Annals of the Caliphs' Kitchens* (an English translation of Ibn Sayyar al-Warraq's tenth-century Baghdadi cookbook).

HENRY NOTAKER graduated from the University of Oslo with a degree in literature and worked for many years as a foreign correspondent and host of arts and letters shows on Norwegian national television. He has written several books about food history, and with *Food Culture in Scandinavia* he won the Gourmand World Cookbook Award for best culinary history in 2009. His last book is a bibliography of early-modern culinary literature, *Printed Cookbooks in Europe 1470–1700*. He is a member of the editorial board of the journal *Food and History*.

KELLY O' LEARY is a graduate student at Boston University in gastronomy and food studies and executive chef at the Bayridge University Residence and Cultural Center.

FABIO PARASECOLI is associate professor and coordinator of food studies at the New School in New York City. He is author of *Food Culture in Italy* (2004) and *Bite Me: Food and Popular Culture* (2008).

SUSAN JI-YOUNG PARK is the program director and head of curriculum development at École de Cuisine Pasadena; project leader for Green Algeria, a national environmental initiative; and a writer for LAWEEKLY'S Squid Ink. She has written curriculum for cooking classes at Los Angeles Unified School District, Sur La Table, Whole Foods Market, Central Market, and Le Cordon Bleu North America. She and her husband, Chef Farid Zadi, have cowritten recipes for *Gourmet Magazine* and the *Los Angeles Times*. The couple are currently writing several cookbooks on North African, French, and Korean cuisines.

ROSEMARY PARKINSON is author of *Culinaria: The Caribbean, Nyam Jamaica*, and *Barbados Bu'n-Bu'n*, and she contributes culinary travel stories to Caribbean magazines.

CHARLES PERRY majored in Middle East languages at Princeton University, the University of California, Berkeley, and the Middle East Centre for Arab Studies, Shimlan, Lebanon. From 1968 to 1976 he was a copy editor and staff writer at *Rolling Stone* magazine in San Francisco, before leaving to work as a freelance writer specializing in food. From 1990 to 2008, he was a staff writer in the food section of the *Los Angeles Times*. He has published widely on the history of Middle Eastern food and was a major contributor to the *Oxford Companion to Food* (1999).

IRINA PETROSIAN is a native of Armenia and a professional journalist who has written for Russian, Armenian, and U.S.-based newspapers. She is the coauthor of *Armenian Food: Fact, Fiction, and Folklore* and holds degrees in journalism from Moscow State University and Indiana University.

SUZANNE PISCOPO is a nutrition, family, and consumer studies lecturer at the University of Malta in Malta. She is mainly involved in the training of home economics and primary-level teachers, as well as in nutrition and consumer-education projects in different settings. Suzanne is a registered public health nutritionist, and her research interests focus on socioecological determinants of food intake, nutrition interventions, and health promotion. She has also written a series of short stories for children about food. Suzanne enjoys teaching and learning about the history and culture of food and is known to creatively experiment with the ingredients at hand when cooking the evening meal together with her husband, Michael.

THERESA PRESTON-WERNER is an advanced graduate student in anthropology at Northwestern University.

MEG RAGLAND is a culinary history researcher and librarian. She lives in Boston, Massachusetts.

CAROL SELVA RAJAH is an award-winning chef and food writer currently based in Sydney, Australia. She has written ten cookbooks on Malaysian and Southeast Asian cuisine. Her book *The Food of India* won the gold award for the Best Hardcover Recipe Book at the prestigious Jacob's Creek World Food Media Awards.

BIRGIT RICQUIER is pursuing a PhD in linguistics at the Université Libre de Bruxelles and the Royal Museum for Central Africa, Tervuren, Belgium, with a fellowship from the Fonds de la Recherche Scientifique (FNRS). The topic of her PhD project is "A Comparative Linguistic Approach to the History of Culinary Practice in Bantu-Speaking Africa." She has spent several months in central Africa, including one month in the Democratic Republic of the Congo as a member of the Boyekoli Ebale Congo 2010 Expedition and two months of research focused on food cultures in Congo.

AMY RIOLO is an award-winning author, lecturer, cooking instructor, and consultant. She is the author of *Arabian Delights: Recipes and Princely*

Entertaining Ideas from the Arabian Peninsula, Nile Style: Egyptian Cuisine and Culture, and *The Mediterranean Diabetes Cookbook*. Amy has lived, worked, and traveled extensively through Egypt and enjoys fusing cuisine, culture, and history into all aspects of her work.

OWEN ROBERTS is a journalist, communications instructor, and director of research communications for the University of Guelph in Guelph, Ontario, Canada. He holds a doctorate of education from Texas Tech University and Texas A&M University.

FIONA ROSS is a gastrodetective whose headquarters is the Bodleian Library in Oxford, United Kingdom. She spends her time there investigating the eating foibles of the famous and infamous. Her cookery book *Dining with Destiny* is the result: when you want to know what Lenin lunched on or what JFK ate by the poolside, *Dining with Destiny* has the answer.

SIGNE ROUSSEAU (née Hansen) is Danish by birth but a long-term resident of southern Africa and is a researcher and part-time lecturer at the University of Cape Town. Following an MA in the Department of English and a PhD (on food media and celebrity chefs) in the Centre for Film and Media Studies, she now teaches critical literacy and professional communication in the School of Management Studies (Faculty of Commerce).

KATHLEEN RYAN is a consulting scholar in the African Section of the University of Pennsylvania Museum of Archaeology and Anthropology, Philadelphia. She has carried out research in Kenya since 1990, when she began a study of Maasai cattle herders in Kajiado District.

HELEN SABERI was Alan Davidson's principal assistant in the completion of the *Oxford Companion to Food*. She is the author of *Noshe Djan: Afghan Food and Cookery;* coauthor of *Trifle* with Alan Davidson; and coauthor of *The Road to Vindaloo* with David Burnett; her latest book is *Tea: A Global History*.

CARI SÁNCHEZ holds a master of arts in gastronomy from the University of Adelaide/Le Cordon Bleu in South Australia. Her dissertation explores the global spread of the Argentine *asado*. She currently lives in Jacksonville, Florida, where she writes the food and travel blog *viCARIous* and is the marketing manager for a craft brewery.

PETER SCHOLLIERS teaches history at the Vrije Universiteit Brussel and is currently head of the research group "Social and Cultural Food Studies" (FOST). He studies the history of food in Europe in the nineteenth and twentieth centuries. He coedits the journal *Food and History* and is involved in various ways in the Institut Européen d'Histoire et des Cultures de l'Alimentation (Tours, France). Recently, he published *Food Culture in Belgium* (Greenwood, 2008). More information can be found at http://www.vub.ac.be/FOST/fost_in_english/.

COLLEEN TAYLOR SEN is the author of *Food Culture in India; Curry: A Global History; Pakoras, Paneer, Pappadums: A Guide to Indian Restaurant Menus*, and many articles on the food of the Indian Subcontinent. She is a regular participant in the Oxford Food Symposium.

ROGER SERUNYIGO was born and lives in Kampala, Uganda. He graduated from Makerere University with a degree in urban and regional planning, has worked in telecommunications, and is now a professional basketball player for the Uganda National Team. He also coaches a women's basketball team (the Magic Stormers).

DORETTE SNOVER is a chef and author. Influenced by French heritage and the food traditions of the Pennsylvania Dutch country, Chef Snover teaches exploration of the world via a culinary map at her school, C'est si Bon! in Chapel Hill. While the stock simmers, she is writing a novel about a French bread apprentice.

CELIA SORHAINDO is a freelance photographer and writer. She was the editor of the 2008 and 2009 *Dominica Food and Drink Guide* magazine and content manager for the Dominica section of the magazine *Caribbean Homes & Lifestyle*.

LYRA SPANG is a PhD candidate in the Department of Anthropology and the Food Studies Program at Indiana University. She has written about food, sex, and symbolism; the role of place in defining organic; and the importance of social relationships in small-scale food business in Belize. She grew up on a farm in southern Belize and is a proud promoter of that country's unique and diverse culinary heritage.

LOIS STANFORD is an agricultural anthropologist in the Department of Anthropology at New Mexico State University. In her research, she has examined the globalization of food systems both in Mexico and in the U.S. Southwest. Her current research focuses on the critical role of food heritage and plant conservation in constructing and maintaining traditional foodways and cultural identity in New Mexico. In collaboration with local food groups, she is currently developing a community food assessment project in the Mesilla Valley in southern New Mexico.

ALIZA STARK is a senior faculty member at the Agriculture, Food, and Environment Institute of Biochemistry, Food Science, and Nutrition at the Hebrew University of Jerusalem.

MARIA "GING" GUTIERREZ STEINBERG is a marketing manager for a New York City–based specialty food company and a food writer. She has a master's degree in food studies from New York University and is a graduate of Le Cordon Bleu. Her articles have appeared in various publications in Asia and the United States.

ANITA STEWART is a cookbook author and Canadian culinary activist from Elora, Ontario, Canada.

EMILY STONE has written about Guatemalan cuisine in the *Radcliffe Culinary Times*, and she is at work on a nonfiction book about chocolate in Central America. She currently teaches journalism and creative writing at Sun Yat-sen University in Guangzhou, China.

ASELE SURINA is a Russian native and former journalist who now works as a translator and interpreter. Since 1999 she has worked at the Institute of Classical Archaeology at the University of Texas on joint projects with an archaeological museum in Crimea, Ukraine.

AYLIN ÖNEY TAN is an architect by training and studied conservation of historic structures in Turkey, Italy, and the United Kingdom. Eventually, her passion for food and travel led her to write on food. Since 2003, she has had a weekly food column in *Cumhuriyet*, a prestigious national daily, and contributes to various food magazines. She was a jury member of the Slow Food Award 2000–2003, with her nominees receiving awards. She contributes to the Terra Madre and Presidia projects as the leader of the Ankara Convivium. She won the Sophie Coe Award on food history in 2008 for her article "Poppy: Potent yet Frail," presented previously at the Oxford Symposium on Food and Cookery where she's become a regular presenter. Currently, she is the curator of the Culinary Culture Section of Princess Islands' City Museum. She is happy to unite her expertise in archaeology and art history from her previous career with her unbounded interest in food culture.

NICOLE TARULEVICZ teaches at the School of Asian Languages and Studies at the University of Tasmania.

KAREN LAU TAYLOR is a freelance food writer and consultant whose food curriculum vitae includes a master's degree in food studies from New York University, an advanced certificate from the Wine and Spirits Education Trust, and a gig as pastry cook at a five-star hotel after completing L'Academie de Cuisine's pastry arts program. She is working toward a master's degree in public health while she continues to write, teach, test recipes, eat, and drink from her home in Alexandria, Virginia.

THY TRAN is trained as a professional chef. She established Wandering Spoon to provide cooking classes, culinary consultation, and educational programming for culinary academies and nonprofit organizations throughout Northern California. Currently, she is a chef instructor at the International Culinary Schools at the Art Institute of California, San Francisco and Tante Marie's. She is also the founder and director of the Asian Culinary Forum. She coauthored *The Essentials of Asian Cooking, Taste of the World*, and the award-winning guide, *Kitchen Companion*.

LEENA TRIVEDI-GRENIER is a Bay-area food writer, cooking teacher, and social media consultant. Her writings have appeared in *The Business of Food: Encyclopedia of the Food and Drink Industry, Culinary Trends* magazine, and the *Cultural Arts Resources for Teachers and Students* newsletter and will be featured in several upcoming titles by Greenwood Press. She also runs a food/travel/gastronomy blog called *Leena Eats This Blog* (http://www.leenaeats .com).

KARIN VANEKER has written for numerous Dutch newspapers and magazines, specializing in trends and the cultural and other histories of ingredients and cuisines, and has published several books. Furthermore, Vaneker has worked for museums and curated an exhibition about New World taro (L. *Xanthosoma* spp.). At present she is researching its potential in domestic cuisines and gastronomy.

PENNY VAN ESTERIK is professor of anthropology at York University, Toronto, where she teaches nutritional anthropology, advocacy anthropology, and feminist theory. She does fieldwork in Southeast Asia and has developed materials on breast-feeding and women's work and infant and young child feeding.

RICHARD WILK is professor of anthropology and gender studies at Indiana University, where he directs the Food Studies Program. With a PhD in anthropology from the University of Arizona, he has taught at the University of California, Berkeley; University of California, Santa Cruz; New Mexico State University; and University College London and has held fellowships at Gothenburg University and the University of London. His publications include more than 125 papers and book chapters, a textbook in economic anthropology, and several edited volumes. His most recent books are *Home Cooking in the Global Village* (Berg Publishers), *Off the Edge: Experiments in Cultural Analysis* (with Orvar Lofgren; Museum Tusculanum Press), *Fast Food/Slow Food* (Altamira Press), and *Time, Consumption, and Everyday Life* (with Elizabeth Shove and Frank Trentmann; Berg Publishers).

CHELSIE YOUNT is a PhD student of anthropology at Northwestern University in Evanston, Illinois. She lived in Senegal in 2005 and again in 2008, when performing ethnographic research for her master's thesis at the École des Hautes Études en Sciences Sociales in Paris, on the topic of Senegalese food and eating habits.

MARCIA ZOLADZ is a cook, food writer, and food-history researcher with her own Web site, Cozinha da Marcia (Marcia's Kitchen; http://www.cozinhadamarcia.com.br). She is a regular participant and contributor at the Oxford Symposium on Food and History and has published three books in Brazil, Germany, and Holland—*Cozinha Portuguesa* (Portuguese cooking), *Muito Prazer* (Easy recipes), and *Brigadeiros e Bolinhas* (Sweet and savory Brazilian finger foods).

Index